October, 31, 1982 - San Francisco.

To my friend, Bill Slough, with best wishes,

Henry M. Clayman, M.D.

October, 31, 1982 - San Francisco.

Intraocular lens implantation
TECHNIQUES AND COMPLICATIONS

Intraocular lens implantation
TECHNIQUES AND COMPLICATIONS

HENRY M. CLAYMAN, M.D.

Clinical Associate Professor of Ophthalmology,
Bascom Palmer Eye Institute,
University of Miami School of Medicine;
Clinical Professor of Health Sciences,
Miami-Dade Community College, Miami, Florida

NORMAN S. JAFFE, M.D.

Clinical Professor of Ophthalmology,
Bascom Palmer Eye Institute,
University of Miami School of Medicine, Miami;
Chairman, Department of Ophthalmology,
St. Francis Hospital, Miami Beach, Florida

MILES A. GALIN, M.D.

Professor of Ophthalmology,
New York Medical College,
New York, New York

with 428 illustrations

The C. V. Mosby Company

ST. LOUIS • TORONTO • LONDON   1983

MOSBY

A TRADITION OF PUBLISHING EXCELLENCE

Editor: Eugenia A. Klein
Assistant editors: Kathryn H. Falk, Jean F. Carey
Manuscript editor: Stephen Dierkes
Book design: Kay M. Kramer
Production: Susan Trail

The C.V. Mosby Company
11830 Westline Industrial Drive, St. Louis, Missouri 63141

Library of Congress Cataloging in Publication Data

Clayman, Henry M.
    Intraocular lens implantation: techniques and complications.

    Bibliography: p.
    Includes index.
    1. Intraocular lenses. I. Jaffe, Norman S.,
1924-   . II. Galin, Miles A. III. Title.
[DNLM: 1. Lenses, Intraocular—Atlases. WW 17
C622i]
RE988.C58 1982   617.7'524   82-8267
ISBN 0-8016-1080-X

GW/CB/B 9 8 7 6 5 4 3 2 1   05/A/630

Preface

No one doubts that the quality of vision obtained with an intraocular lens implantation more closely resembles that of the phakic eye than the vision obtained by any other known method. However, because intraocular lens implant surgery is more complex than a routine cataract extraction, its history has been exciting, often frustrating, but finally rewarding. There have been abortive attempts at intraocular lens implantation dating back to the early eighteenth century, but it was not until 1967 that ophthalmic surgeons in the United States began performing implant surgery in appreciable numbers. Although implant surgery is not an American innovation, the United States has become the central stage for it.

We recognized early the efficacy of intraocular lens implantation and were confident of its future wide popularity and acceptance. This conviction sustained us during the years of formidable professional and bureaucratic opposition. What we did not predict was the evolution of cataract extraction and lens implantation. The intracapsular method is steadily being replaced by the extracapsular method, and the lens implants that failed terribly in the 1950s and early 1960s are now the most popular lenses in use, albeit in modified designs.

Several factors have contributed to the evolution of lens implant surgery. First there was the introduction of phacoemulsification, a technique of cataract extraction initially irrelevant to intraocular lenses, whose great advantages were a small incision and rapid patient rehabilitation. As an aside, phacoemulsification was a variant of extracapsular cataract extraction, and the profession slowly became aware of certain panocular benefits of this type of surgery. In the meantime, the European pioneers were the pacesetters for the United States, and they inspired the widespread popularity of the iris-fixated intraocular lenses with which their names are associated. The exception was Choyce, whose lens was angle fixated. Although iris-supported lenses now appear headed for certain obsolescence, we must be grateful for their introduction. They rescued the field of lens implantation from a tragic experience and created a revival of enthusiasm for this procedure.

In the middle 1970s most implant surgeons in the United States were using intracapsular cataract extraction techniques and iris-fixated intraocular lenses. This combination did not satisfy all the patient requirements of rapid visual rehabilitation and unrestricted life-style, nor was it suitable for all patients. Furthermore, the necessity of coping with a bulging anterior hyaloid face and placing a fixation suture or bending a fixation clip sometimes turned a routine cataract extraction into a formidable surgical exercise. How much easier it was to slide an anterior chamber lens into the anterior chamber, instead of contending with iris retraction in the face of positive vitreous pressure. It was for this reason that the interest in anterior chamber lenses grew—in other words, the profession evolved a lens type that simplified the surgery and hence benefited the patient.

Analogous to this was the situation with posterior chamber intraocular lenses. When Shearing introduced his lens in late 1977, the perfect match was made between phacoemulsification and an intraocular lens which required an extracapsular technique. This uniplanar lens could be inserted through a modestly enlarged phacoemulsification incision, without the anterior chamber collapsing because its uniplanar design easily slipped through the incision without prying it apart. Moreover, implant length was not a factor, as in anterior chamber lens implants. Of course, there were surgeons performing routine extracapsular cataract surgery, without emulsification, who were using two-plane intraocular lenses of the Binkhorst iridocapsular and Worst Platina type. Implant insertion is considerably easier with Shearing-type posterior chamber lenses, and fixation is better; these extracapsular cataract surgeons slowly gravitated to posterior chamber lenses. Why? Because it was the type of lens that simplified surgery. Concurrently, medical instrumentation was improving with the development of better and more versatile microscopes and automated techniques of extracapsular surgery.

Where is this taking us? We feel that the drift is to extracapsular cataract surgery and specifically to small incision surgery such as phacoemulsification, with the insertion of uniplanar intraocular lenses capable of being introduced through a relatively small incision. Because the length of anterior chamber lenses is an added intraoperative factor to consider, we believe that posterior chamber intraocular lenses will slowly gain the favor of the majority of surgeons. The advantage of small-incision cataract surgery with uniplanar intraocular lens implantation for rapid patient physical and visual rehabilitation is obvious, but the ultimate expression of minimum patient inconvenience and minimum disruption of patient life-style is the astonishing growth of outpatient cataract surgery. With promising laser techniques on the horizon, noninvasive cataract surgery may be feasible.

Progress in cataract surgery and intraocular lens implantation over the past 30 years has been astonishing. Rapid physical and visual rehabilitation has become almost routine. Yet, the details of technique are increasing at a rapid pace. This atlas describes the principles underlying these techniques and is based on our years of experience. We do not describe every technique, nor every lens, nor every complication.

Henry M. Clayman
Norman S. Jaffe
Miles A. Galin

Contents

One

Techniques of cataract extraction

GENERAL PRINCIPLES

The purpose of this chapter is to give methods by which a safe intracapsular cataract extraction (ICCE), extracapsular cataract extraction (ECCE), or Kelman phacoemulsification (KPE) can be performed on the premise that an intraocular lens (IOL) will then be inserted. The variations in techniques and instrumentation are numerous, and we make no attempt to describe them all. We present examples of methods that we have found safe and effective. Our omission of a specific procedure or instrument is not intended to reflect unfavorably on ophthalmic surgeons whose views may differ from ours. Furthermore, we are avoiding a discussion of anesthesia in ophthalmic surgery, since the reader will find this covered by sources cited in the bibliography. All maneuvers are described with the assumption that the surgeon is right-handed.

Operating microscope

Before detailing the various types of cataract surgery, we wish to state unequivocally that the surgery described in this atlas requires the use of the operating microscope. The surgeon may have to use both hands simultaneously and for this reason would desire a foot-controlled microscope. At the time of this writing the Zeiss Op Mi6 or 6S with "X-Y" motion is our choice for the performance of sophisticated anterior segment surgery.

Prior to the cataract operation by whatever methods, there are several common considerations. The first is the concept of surgery on the "soft eye," which is of paramount importance in intracapsular cataract surgery and becomes less important as one moves to extracapsular cataract surgery and then to phacoemulsification. One might say that the topic becomes less crucial as the incision gets smaller; nevertheless it is always important. Methods of producing a soft eye include digital pressure, ocular compression by balloon de-

1

vices, hyperosmotic agents, and carbonic anhydrase inhibitors—each alone or in combination. We shall assume that the eye has a satisfactory intraocular pressure commensurate with the procedure being undertaken, prior to the start of the operation. Next is the selection of lid retractors of which there are many types. We recommend the Jaffe lid retractors (Fig. 1-1), which are sufficiently adjustable and malleable to conform to any peculiarity of the patient's physiognomy.

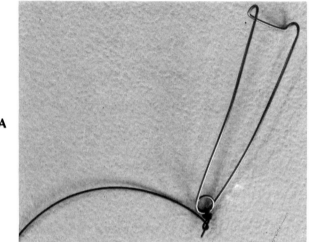

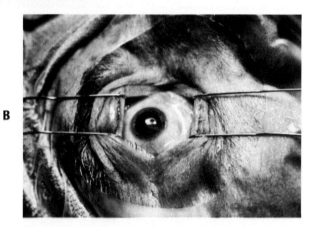

Fig. 1-1. A, Jaffe lid retractor. **B,** Jaffe lid retractor in situ. (From Jaffe, N.S.: Cataract surgery and its complications, ed. 3, St. Louis, 1981, The C.V. Mosby Co.)

Superior rectus suture

A superior rectus suture should be used to rotate the eye as required; this may be placed transconjunctivally or under the conjunctival flap. In the former method the globe is rotated down and slightly posteriorly. With toothed forceps (e.g., Lester forceps) held in the left hand, conjunctiva, Tenon's capsule, and superior rectus muscle are grasped at the 12 o'clock position approximately 10 mm posterior to the limbus. A 4-0 silk suture is then passed beneath them and out through the conjunctiva (Fig. 1-2). This maneuver is aided by slightly lifting the forceps held in the left hand. The correct placement of the suture is ascertained by pulling it inferiorly, whereupon the globe should rotate downward. In a deep-set eye with a fornix-based conjunctival flap, it may be prudent to place the superior rectus suture under the flap, thus retracting the conjunctiva with the traction suture and enhancing exposure. In this case the forceps held in the left hand are passed under the flap, the tendon of the superior rectus muscle is grasped, and the globe rotated downward. The suture is then passed under the muscle insertion. In either method the long ends of the suture are kept out of the operative field by being looped under the nasal arm of the superior lid retractor.

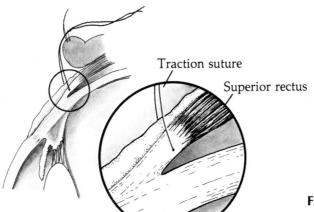

Traction suture

Superior rectus

Fig. 1-2. Superior rectus suture.

Conjunctival flap

We will assume that the surgeon will perform either a fornix- or limbal-based conjunctival flap. The former (Fig. 1-3) is performed by grasping the conjunctiva and Tenon's capsule with fine-toothed forceps at the limbus and "buttonholing" it with Westcott scissors to the bare sclera. The *closed* scissors are then passed laterally through the buttonhole to the left under the conjunctiva and Tenon's capsule following their limbal insertion. The scissors are opened, which lyses the adhesions of Tenon's capsule to the sclera. The scissors are then withdrawn and reinserted with the proximal blade under the conjunctiva and Tenon's capsule at their limbal insertion and the other blade over the insertion. When the scissors are closed, a neat fornix-based flap without tags will result. This maneuver is continued to the right and left depending on the size flap required, which in turn will depend on the operative procedure contemplated. Lateral incisions at the extremities of the flap are options that will permit the flap to be retracted further posteriorly.

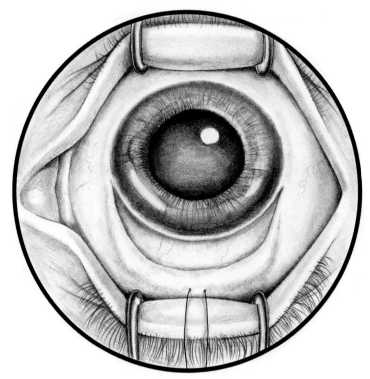

Fig. 1-3. Fornix-based conjunctival flap.

A limbus-based flap (Fig. 1-4) varies in width from 2 to 7 mm. The conjunctiva is grasped at the 12 o'clock position in the line of incision with a fine-toothed forceps held in the left hand and tented upward. It is then incised to the sclera with Westcott scissors. As in the fornix-based conjunctival flap, closed scissors are passed through the opening laterally in the line of incision and opened to lyse adhesions. The scissors are withdrawn and reinserted with the distal blade under the conjunctiva and Tenon's capsule. The scissors are closed, which results in a clean, curvilinear edge to the flap margin. Again the size of the flap depends on the proposed operation. Dissection of the flap to the limbus can be continued with fine microscissors and the limbus exposed with a no. 64 Beaver blade, although numerous other instruments can be used.

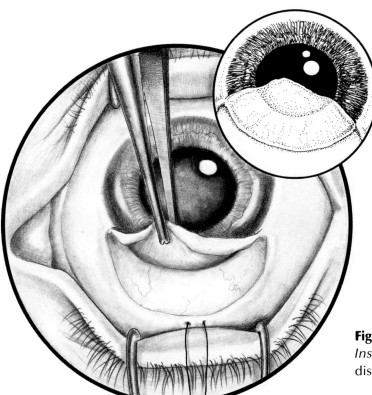

Fig. 1-4. Limbus-based conjunctival flap. *Inset,* Limbus-based conjunctival flap after dissection.

In both types of flaps the dissection is often facilitated by ballooning the superior conjunctiva with a balanced saline or anesthetic solution. Bleeding is contained with the wet field cautery (Fig. 1-5), and further hemostasis may be obtained with cellulose sponges soaked in epinephrine (1:1000) pressed gently on the limbus. Care should be taken not to press the sponges on the cornea since they leave an imprint, thus detracting from the surgeon's view of the anterior chamber—an undesirable situation when an IOL is planned.

At the conclusion of the procedure a fornix-based flap is pulled down over the incision and will often adhere to its original insertion; or it may be tacked at its extremity to the adjacent conjunctiva with one or two absorbable sutures such as 8-0 Vicryl. The flap should overlap the incision by about 1 or 2 mm and will usually retract back to the limbus within 4 weeks after the operation. A limbal-based flap is pulled back over the incision and sutured to the adjacent conjunctiva with an absorbable suture. Even with the 180-degree limbal-based flap, rarely are more than four sutures required for closure. A very small limbal-based flap such as in phacoemulsification often requires no suture. It is laid back over the incision and is adherent the next day. An alternative to suturing the conjunctival flap is to use a wet field cautery with coaptation forceps. This method works, although conjunctiva to conjunctiva adhesion may be short lived.

The advantages of a limbal-based flap are that the incision is well covered and a "handle" to elevate the cornea is provided. The disadvantages are that it obscures visualization during IOL insertion (especially with intracameral iris sutures (p. 219), and the corneal-scleral sutures frequently draw Tenon's capsule of the flap into the tract during suturing. Furthermore, in the postoperative period it is easier to cut sutures under a fornix-based flap should this be necessary to reduce with-the-rule astigmatism.

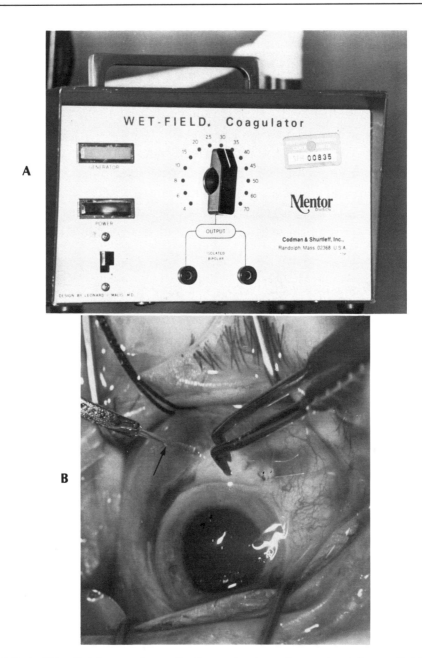

Fig. 1-5. **A,** Wet field coagulator. **B,** Cauterization of vessels with wet field cautery. Note stream of balanced saline solution *(arrow),* which acts as dielectric between jaws of bipolar forceps.

INTRACAPSULAR CATARACT EXTRACTION
Incision

The literature on the placement of the corneal scleral incision is copious and there is no agreement on the site, on the amount of beveling, or about whether the incision should be uniplanar or multiplanar. The topic is partially summarized by stating that the more corneal the section the more the astigmatism, and the more scleral the section the greater the risk of hyphema. Figs. 1-6 and 1-7 show two views of a uniplanar incision of moderate bevel placed in the surgical limbus. A razor knife is used for the initial incision. A razor knife is sharp on only one side and therefore, if it is applied perpendicularly to the sclera, a blunt and sharp edge are simultaneously present and

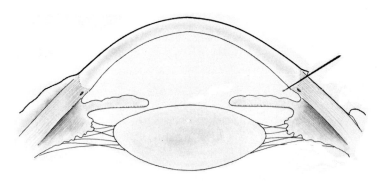

Fig. 1-6. Uniplanar incision showing angulation.

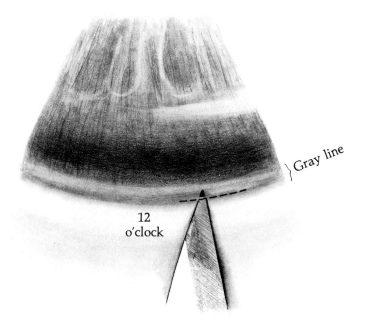

Fig. 1-7. Placement of incision with razor knife in posterior third of surgical limbus.

scleral penetration may be difficult. A better method is to grasp the sclera at the 12 o'clock position just posterior to the limbus with a 0.12-mm toothed forceps held in the left hand and to present the razor edge to the sclera slightly obliquely with the sharp edge to the surgeon's right. Gentle pressure is exerted with the knife as it is swung to a perpendicular angle, and the blade will enter the anterior chamber with ease. While the blade is still in the anterior chamber, it is used to extend the incision 4 mm to the right, in the line of the surgical limbus, so that the corneal-scleral section scissors can be introduced. The incision is enlarged to the right to the 9:30 position following the surgical limbus and to the left to the 2:30 position (Fig. 1-8). This will give a 170-degree section (Fig. 1-9) almost corneal at its lateral aspects, which is de-

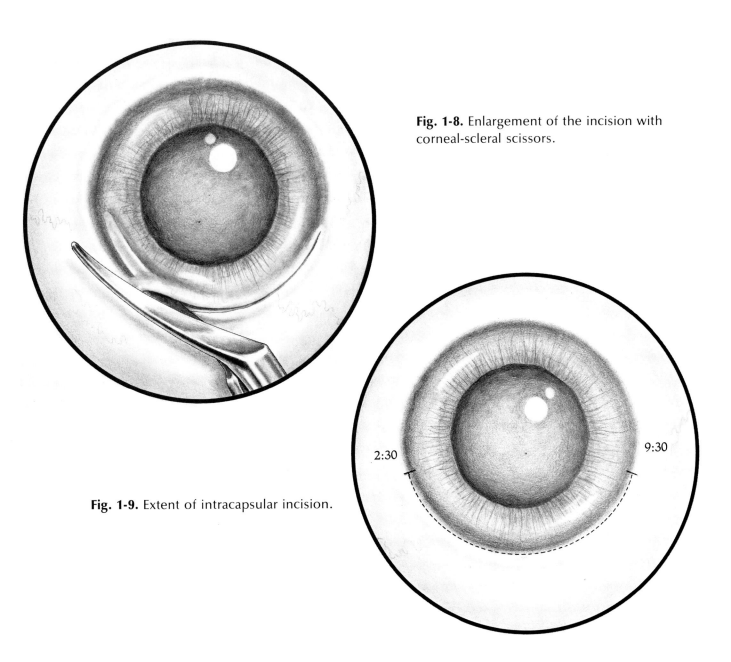

Fig. 1-8. Enlargement of the incision with corneal-scleral scissors.

Fig. 1-9. Extent of intracapsular incision.

2:30

9:30

sirable to prevent bleeding from the long, perforating, lateral blood vessels (Fig. 1-10), and also to minimize with-the-rule astigmatism, monotonously produced when interrupted monofilament sutures are used to close the incision. A safety suture (e.g., 8-0 Vicryl) is placed at the 12 o'clock position through both the corneal and scleral aspects of the incision and looped to the surgeon's left.

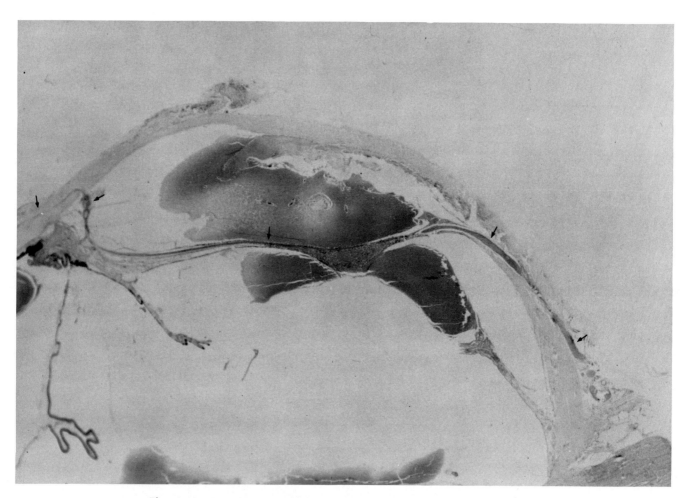

Fig. 1-10. Fortuitous pathology section showing course of long ciliary nerve and vessels *(arrows).*

Jaffe-Barraquer scissors (Fig. 1-11, *A*) will give a beveled biplane incision even if the initial incision was uniplanar. Clayman-Troutman scissors (Fig. 1-11, *B*), which are also calibrated, will give a single-plane incision when the blades are perpendicular to the sclera. If the surgeon tips his hand posteriorly and presents the blades obliquely to the sclera, a biplane incision will result.

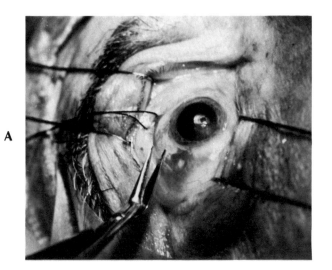

A

Fig. 1-11. A, Jaffe-Barraquer scissors. **B,** Calibrated Clayman-Troutman scissors. (**A** from Jaffe, N.S.: Cataract surgery and its complications, ed. 3, St. Louis, 1981, The C.V. Mosby Co.; **B** courtesy Storz Instrument Co.)

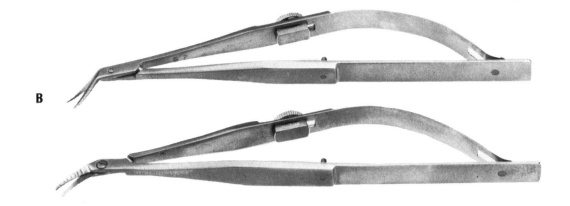

B

Peripheral iridectomy

One or more peripheral iridectomies (or iridotomies) are performed (Fig. 1-12, *A*). Fig. 1-12, *B* and *C*, shows the iris being grasped with forceps held in the left hand while a knuckle of iris is excised with microscissors held in the right hand. In the illustration the scissors are angled laterally, which will result in a broad-based peripheral iridectomy. If the scissors are angled vertically, a narrower, pie-shaped peripheral iridectomy will result. In either case care should be taken to avoid snipping the ciliary process because this results in hemorrhage.

As stated at the beginning of the chapter, we wish to present a technique compatible with IOL implantation. To accomplish this, additional iris surgery may be necessary (p. 197).

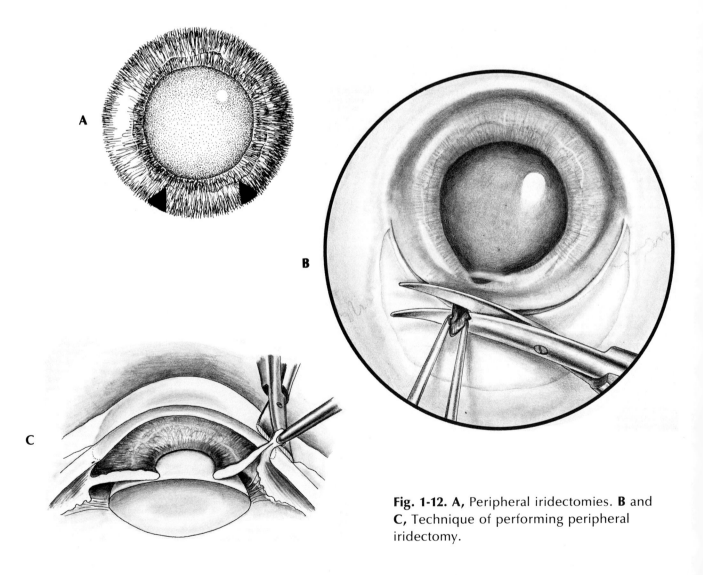

Fig. 1-12. A, Peripheral iridectomies. **B** and **C,** Technique of performing peripheral iridectomy.

Cryoextraction of the cataract

Prior to cataract extraction many surgeons inject intracameral α-chymotrypsin to effect enzymatic zonulolysis, although this is probably redundant in older patients. The cornea is then elevated by means of the 12 o'clock safety suture, and the anterior chamber is dried with a cellulose sponge to enhance cryoadhesion. The iris is retracted with Hoskins no. 19 forceps held in the left hand, and the cryoprobe, held in the right hand, is applied to the anterior capsule at the junction of the lower two thirds with the upper one third of the crystalline lens (Fig. 1-13). The probe is activated to produce a medium size ice ball, thus adhering its tip to the underlying anterior capsule and cortex. With a gentle, to-and-fro, lateral rocking motion the lenticular-zonular attachments are broken as the cataract is slowly withdrawn from the posterior chamber (Fig. 1-14), through the pupillary aperture, and out

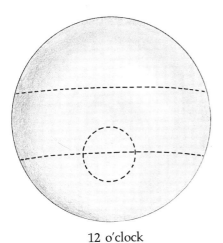

12 o'clock

Fig. 1-13. Position of cryoprobe on cataractous lens.

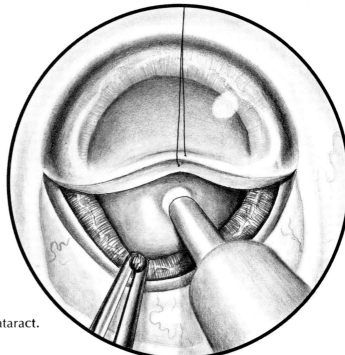

Fig. 1-14. Cryoextraction of cataract.

through the incision. As soon as the lateral poles of the cataract clear the pupillary margin, the iris retraction forceps can be released and the cornea slowly lowered, avoiding endothelial contact to the ice ball. If the cryoprobe is excessively cold, the ice ball will be too big and may adhere to the iris and cornea, precluding cataract extraction. We recommend the 1.5-mm straight cryoprobe; this should be tested prior to use to ensure that it freezes adequately, without an overly large ice ball.

Many surgeons prefer to use a cellulose sponge or an iris retractor to retract the iris as a prelude to cataract extraction. Our preference is for a forceps in the left hand to retract the iris because it gives versatility should an additional surgical maneuver be necessary. For example, the forceps may be used to strip zonules (Figs. 1-15 and 1-16), elevate an inadvertently dropped cornea, or clear a preplaced suture from the field.

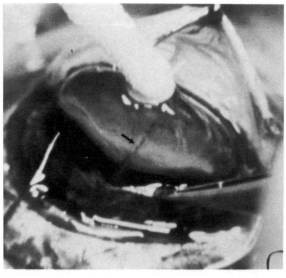

Fig. 1-15. Residual zonules adherent to lens. (From Jaffe, N.S.: Cataract surgery and its complications, ed. 3, St. Louis, 1981, The C.V. Mosby Co.)

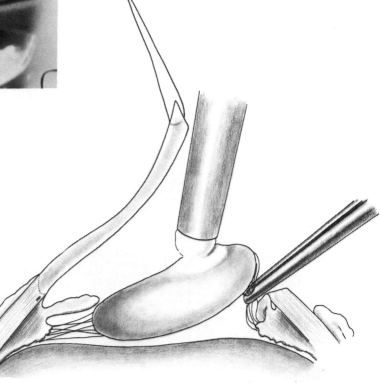

Fig. 1-16. Stripping zonules.

Re-formation of the anterior chamber and suturing

After the cataract is extracted, iris will often be left prolapsing through the incision. This is swept and irrigated back into the anterior chamber (Fig. 1-17). The anterior chamber is then re-formed with air and balanced saline or sodium hyaluronate (p. 272), and the 12 o'clock suture is tied and trimmed.

We will avoid a discussion of preplaced, postplaced, running, and mixed suturing and state that 10-0 nylon, as an interrupted suture, is a reliable closure for the cataract incision. For a 170-degree section we would use seven to nine 10-0 nylon sutures in addition to the 12 o'clock safety suture (Fig. 1-18). The first ''lay-down'' is in three overhand loops (as 10-0 nylon requires)

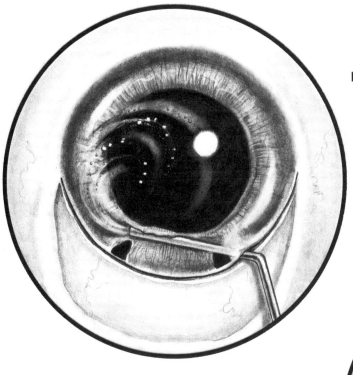

Fig. 1-17. Repositioning prolapsed iris.

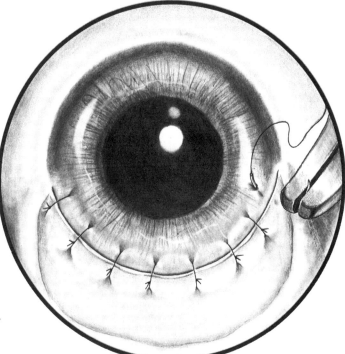

Fig. 1-18. Closure of intracapsular incision.

and is then squared with two separate overhand ties. The suture is trimmed close to the knot but not directly on it, lest it unravel. Some surgeons slip the knot back in the suture tract by traction on the suture. It is easier to bury the knot at the corneal aspect of the incision; therefore the knot is slid anteriorly. The incision is covered by the conjunctival flap as noted previously.

Comment

There are an extraordinary number of variations of ICCE and the technique of Galin is an example. He uses a limbal-based flap and makes an initial vertical groove of one half the scleral thickness for the whole length of the incision in the surgical limbus. He then places three 6-0 silk sutures at 10, 12, and 1 o'clock, respectively, through the margins of the groove. These are swept aside with a spatula to clear the wound for the section. The anterior chamber is entered with a Wheeler knife, and the section is completed to the right and left with Castroviejo blunt-tipped, side-angled keratoplasty scissors giving a two-plane, "mitered" incision. The cornea is elevated by the conjunctival flap, and the cataract is extracted with capsule forceps by tumbling and without α-chymotrypsin. Peripheral iridectomies are performed, and the IOL is inserted in a formed anterior chamber. The preplaced sutures are tied and additional sutures are placed where required. Galin's technique raises an interesting point inasmuch as he favors the Fyodorov Sputnik IOL (p. 119), and this lens requires no intracameral fixation suture. However, when a preplaced iris fixation suture is required (pp. 86 and 99), the additional presence of preplaced corneal-scleral sutures leads to a cluttered field. It is for this reason that we advocate only one 12 o'clock safety suture in the intracapsular technique initially described.

COOPERVISION SYSTEMS/CAVITRON

Kelman phacoemulsification is a variant of ECCE, and we use the equipment of CooperVision Systems/Cavitron* for both procedures. The CooperVision Systems/Cavitron 6000 and 6500 units, being designed for ECCE, have automated irrigation and aspiration. The CooperVision Systems/Cavitron 7007 and 8000 models have an ultrasonic mode in addition to irrigation and aspiration and are suited to both KPE and ECCE. For an ECCE the I/A PAK is used, while the UNIPAK is required for a KPE.

We shall briefly describe the CooperVision Systems/Cavitron 6500 and 8000 models, both of which are activated by a foot pedal once the power is turned on. The CooperVision Systems/Cavitron 6500 is portable and has two foot positions: number 1, irrigation, and number 2, irrigation and aspiration (I/A) (Fig. 1-19). There are two settings in aspiration, I/A MIN (65 mm

---

*CooperVision Systems/Cavitron, Irvine, CA. A detailed description of this equipment may be obtained from the sources cited in the bibliography and from the technical manuals available from CooperVision Systems/Cavitron Corporation.

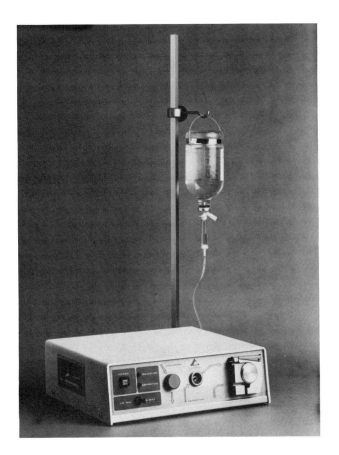

Fig. 1-19. CooperVision Systems/Cavitron Model 6500 (Courtesy CooperVision Systems/Cavitron.)

Hg) and I/A MAX (370 mm Hg). Two handpieces are provided: a unimode irrigation handpiece and a bimode irrigation/aspiration handpiece (Fig. 1-20).

The CooperVision Systems/Cavitron 8000 (Fig. 1-21) is capable of phacoemulsification in addition to irrigation and aspiration. The foot pedal (Fig. 1-22) has three positions: number 1, irrigation, number 2, irrigation and aspiration, and number 3, ultrasonic fragmentation with irrigation and aspiration. To use irrigation the vacuum dial is set at "standby" (Fig. 1-23, *A*), and the pedal is depressed to position 1, the only possible setting in the "standby" mode. I/A MIN and I/A MAX (Fig. 1-23, *B* and *C*) are used with the irrigation/aspiration handpiece, and in either of these modes the foot pedal can be depressed to position 1, irrigation, or position 2, irrigation and aspiration. For phacoemulsification of the nucleus the ultrasonic handpiece (Fig. 1-24) is required, and the vacuum is set at U/S (ultrasound) (Fig. 1-23, *D*). The foot pedal may now be used in position 1, 2, or 3 (irrigation, aspiration with ultrasonic fragmentation). When the U/S mode is used, the aspiration is 41 mm Hg.

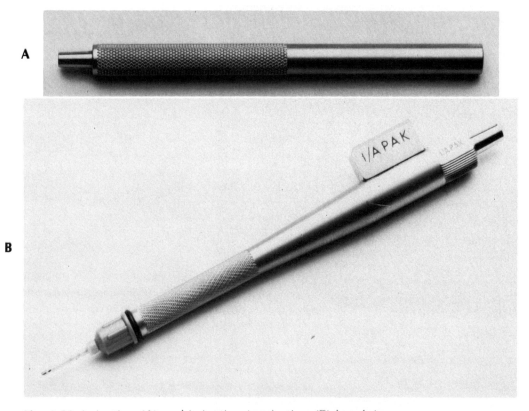

Fig. 1-20. Irrigation **(A)** and irrigation/aspiration **(B)** handpieces. (Courtesy CooperVision Systems/Cavitron.)

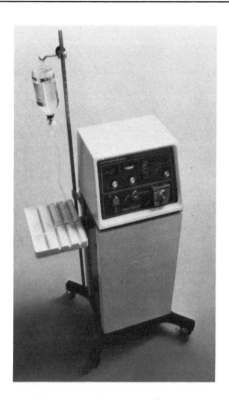

Fig. 1-21. CooperVision Systems/Cavitron Model 8000. (Courtesy CooperVision Systems/Cavitron.)

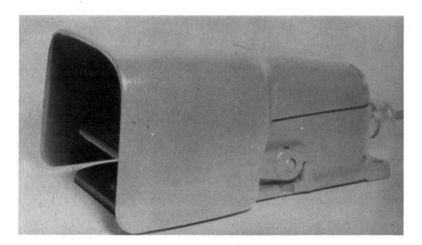

Fig. 1-22. Foot pedal for CooperVision Systems/Cavitron units.

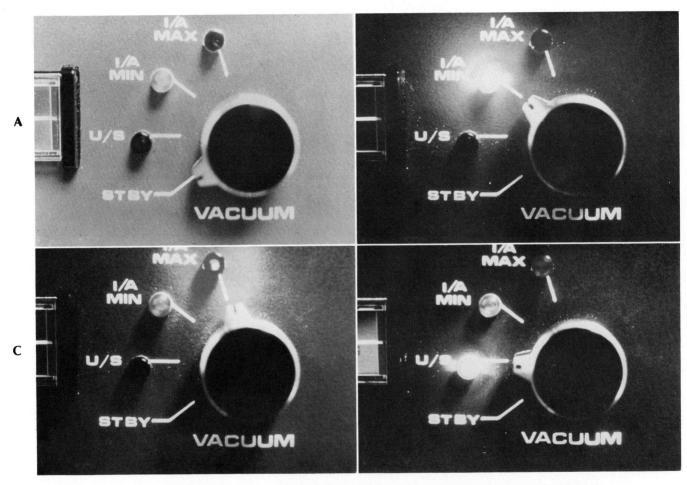

Fig. 1-23. A, Vacuum dial in "standby" mode. **B,** Vacuum dial in I/A minimum mode. **C,** Vacuum dial in I/A maximum mode. **D,** Vacuum dial in ultrasonic mode. (Courtesy CooperVision Systems/Cavitron.)

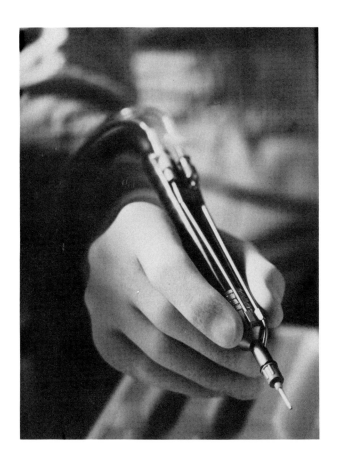

Fig. 1-24. Ultrasonic handpiece. (Courtesy CooperVision Systems/Cavitron.)

EXTRACAPSULAR CATARACT EXTRACTION
Incision

Meticulous positioning of the initial incision is advised for KPE (p. 38); however, an ECCE permits some flexibility, especially in the posterior direction. The 11 o'clock position in the surgical limbus where the anterior two thirds of the limbus meets the posterior one third is a safe and convenient location for a 1.5- to 2-mm incision (Fig. 1-25). This incision may be made more posteriorly, but since the incision is destined to be enlarged, the surgeon is again reminded that hyphemas can be caused by an excessively posterior incision. An extremely anterior incision is not advised primarily because instrumentation may result in corneal damage and secondly because excessive astigmatism may result. The initial incision is made with a razor knife (e.g., Beaver 75L). The incision should not be wedge shaped, since instruments may snag on the inner aspects of the incision. The incision should be squared with the razor knife.

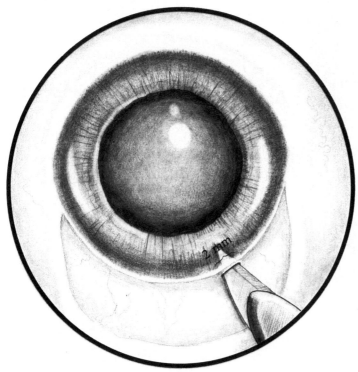

Fig. 1-25. Initial incision for ECCE.

Anterior capsulectomy

Many surgeons use an irrigating cystotome (Fig. 1-26) for this part of the operation. We find that most available instruments of this type lose their sharpness with repeated use and autoclaving, so we favor a disposable 22-gauge needle on which we fashion a small hook at the tip. Specifically the tip of the needle is grasped with a needle holder; care must be taken not to blunt the needle tip. The end of the needle is bent away from the needle orifice so that a 90-degree hook is formed, no more than 1.0 mm in length (Fig. 1-27). The needle/cystotome is then placed on the CooperVision Systems/ Cavitron irrigating handpiece.

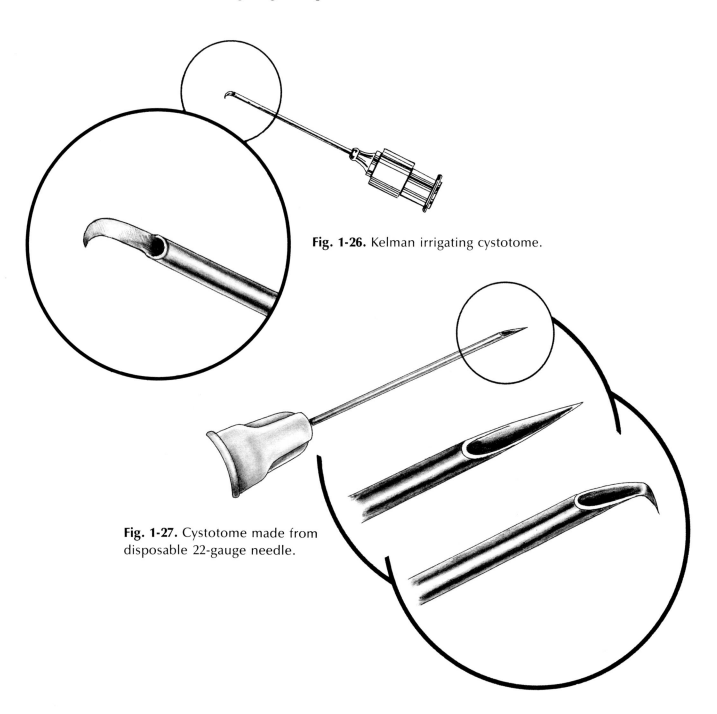

Fig. 1-26. Kelman irrigating cystotome.

Fig. 1-27. Cystotome made from disposable 22-gauge needle.

There are many surgeons who prefer to perform the anterior capsulectomy under air to protect the corneal endothelium; we prefer a closed chamber technique with continuous irrigation for the enhanced visibility. Prior to entering the eye the irrigating handpiece is held vertically with the needle/cystotome pointing upward and the foot pedal depressed until the irrigating solution clears the handpiece and the needle of air. The needle/cystotome is then inserted into the anterior chamber, with the hook horizontal and with continuous irrigation. This maneuver is aided by grasping the anterior lip of the incision with 0.12-mm toothed forceps. Care must be taken to avoid stripping Descemet's membrane or snagging the iris (the latter can cause miosis). Once the hook of the needle has cleared the iris and is in the pupillary space, it is turned from a horizontal position to "point down," i.e., the tip of the hook points posteriorly. Continuous irrigation is maintained and the cornea well irrigated for optimum visualization. The anterior capsule is engaged at the 6 o'clock position just central to the pupillary margin. A series of interconnecting cuts is made concentric to the pupillary margin to form the so-called can-opener capsulectomy (Fig. 1-28, *A* and *B*).

The capsular cuts are made in the plane of the anterior capsule radially, as if they were radiating out from the center of the lens capsule. Ideally the cuts should almost interconnect to avoid pie-shaped pieces of anterior capsular remnants, which have a proclivity to clog the ports of the I/A handpiece during the aspiration phase of the operation. The exact manner in which the capsular cuts are made varies according to which quadrant of the capsule the surgeon is working in. The capsulectomy instrument may be moved backward, forward, or sideway to accomplish a neat anterior capsulectomy without residual tags. We gently pull the needle toward 12 o'clock when we are working in the inferior quadrant and use a rotatory movement in the lateral quadrants. In the superior quadrant the needle is pushed toward the 6 o'clock position. To be more specific, we begin the capsulectomy at the 6 o'clock position and proceed to 12 o'clock. As the capsulectomy is progressively enlarged, the anterior capsule loses its tautness. A looser capsule is more difficult to cut, and tags may be left. It is technically easier to grab and excise a superior tag than an inferior tag (especially with small incision surgery); it is for this reason that we start the capsulectomy at the 6 o'clock position and conclude at 12 o'clock. A completed capsulectomy is analogous to the perforations in a sheet of postage stamps surrounding any given stamp. The surgeon should be able to see the needle tip directly at all times. It is possible to be under the capsule and excoriate the nucleus with the cut and still leave the capsule intact. This is extremely undesirable because a large flap of anterior capsule with a broad attachment is difficult to remove.

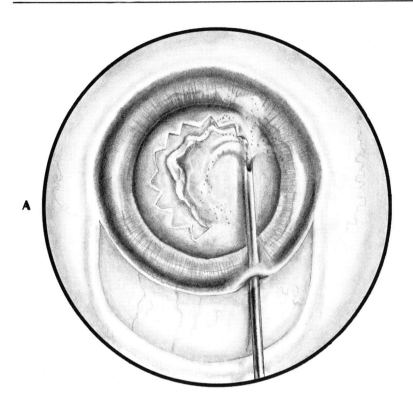

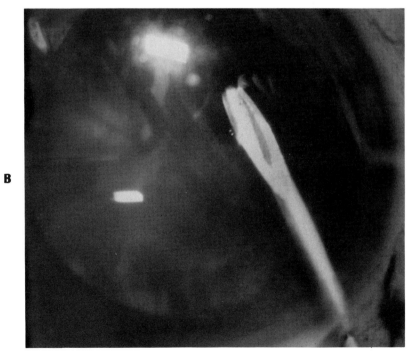

Fig. 1-28. A, "Can-opener" capsulectomy. **B,** Transcorneal visualization of capsulectomy.

Residual capsular tags are more readily seen after the nucleus is removed. If they are significant, they may be removed by inserting Kelman-McPherson forceps through the incision. The capsular tag is then externalized and excised. No attempt to pull capsular tags should be made, since this will tear the capsule posteriorly beyond the equator and result in a posterior capsular defect. A broad-based inferior capsular tag is very difficult to remove, and frequently the best judgment is to leave it alone.

Removal of the nucleus

Removal of the nucleus following the anterior capsulectomy falls into two categories: removing the nucleus from the anterior chamber or removing the nucleus from the posterior chamber.

To remove the nucleus from the anterior chamber, we use the Kelman irrigating cystotome on the CooperVision Systems/Cavitron irrigating handpiece to prolapse the nucleus into the anterior chamber. The cystotome is introduced through the original 2-mm incision under continuous irrigation with the irrigating port facing posteriorly. This washes the iris clear of the cystotome and permits it to be slid into the anterior chamber with minimal iris trauma. Nuclear prolapse is then effected as described under phacoemulsification (p. 39).

The incision is then enlarged (Fig. 1-29) by corneal-scleral section scissors introduced through the initial incision after it has been enlarged to 4 mm with the razor knife. Cut to both the left and right, the section is enlarged to approximately 140 degrees, and an 8-0 Vicryl suture is placed at the 12 o'clock position as described previously (p. 10). If the nucleus was not prolapsed into the anterior chamber and must now be delivered from the posterior chamber, a larger incision of approximately 160 degrees will be required. In either contingency, if the incision appears too small to expel the nucleus, it should be *enlarged.* It is better to have the incision too big than too small.

Once the nucleus is in the anterior chamber, it may be expressed manually or, as we prefer, with the Pearce-Knolle irrigating loop (Fig. 1-30). The loop is attached to the CooperVision Systems/Cavitron irrigating handpiece, and is irrigated free from air. With continuous irrigation the loop is slid under the prolapsed nucleus without corneal retraction. The nucleus is then "shoveled" out of the anterior chamber by the flow of irrigation fluid and the gentle pressure of the irrigating loop on the posterior aspect of the section.

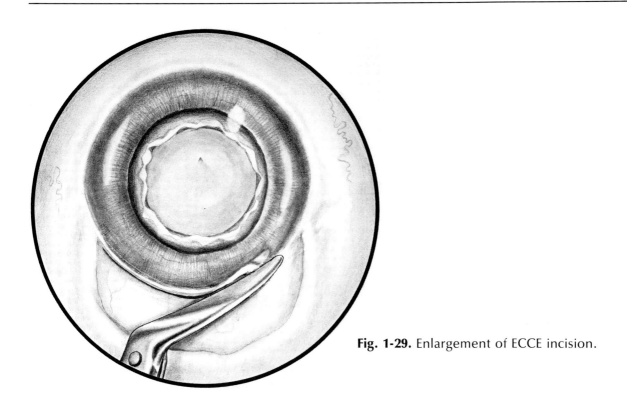

Fig. 1-29. Enlargement of ECCE incision.

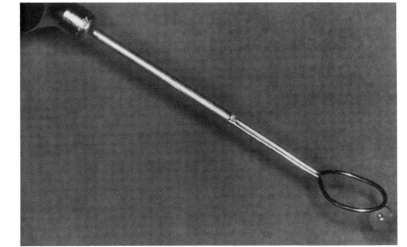

Fig. 1-30. Pearce-Knolle irrigating loop.

When the nucleus is removed from the posterior chamber, we use a lens spoon held in the right hand and a pair of forceps (e.g., Hoskins no. 19) held in the left hand. With an assistant elevating the cornea the iris is retracted with the left hand, exposing the superior pole of the nucleus. The spoon is introduced into the anterior chamber exerting slight posterior pressure on the scleral aspect of the section (Fig. 1-31, *A*). This will cause the superior pole of the nucleus to present itself in an anterior direction. The tip of the spoon can then be slid just *under* the superior pole of the nucleus (see broken arrow, Fig. 1-31, *B*). Gentle, continued posterior pressure on the scleral aspect of the section (often aided by counterpressure on the limbus at the 6 o'clock position by forceps held in the left hand) will cause the nucleus to deliver itself out of the posterior chamber (Fig. 1-31, *C*).

The spoon can be compared to a swimming pool slide. Instead of the swimmer sliding down the slide, imagine the swimmer sliding *up*. The spoon acts as a slide (or guide) for the upward exit of the nucleus from the posterior chamber. It is for this reason that the spoon must be placed *under* the superior pole of the nucleus. A common error is to place it *on* the nucleus, which prevents the nucleus from sliding up the spoon. Continued posterior pressure in this contingency and/or countertraction at the inferior limbus will cause the nucleus to tumble and may rupture the posterior capsule with vitreous loss. If the nucleus appears reluctant to come out, its removal from the posterior chamber can be helped by an assistant spearing it with a fine disposable needle as it appears at the incision.

A special word of caution is directed about cases where pupillary dilatation is inadequate. In these cases the anterior capsulectomy is impeded by the relative miosis. Hence when the iris is retracted to expose the nucleus, the superior pole will be covered by a sheet of capsule. This should be retracted with forceps to facilitate nuclear prolapse. The anterior capsule has a shiny appearance, which distinguishes it from the semimatt appearance of the underlying nucleus.

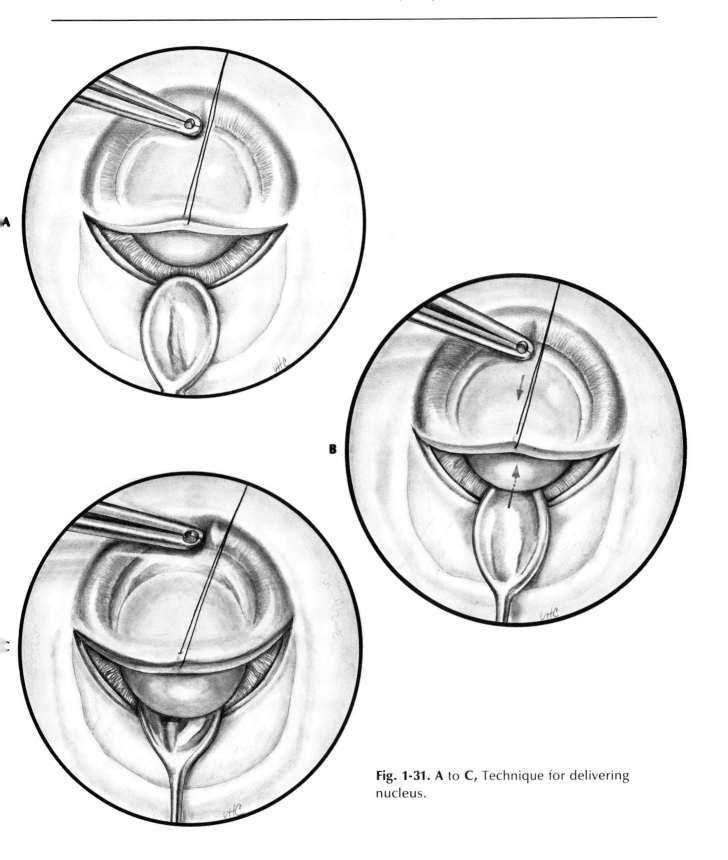

Fig. 1-31. A to **C,** Technique for delivering nucleus.

Closure of the anterior chamber

The next phase is to partially close the anterior chamber so that automated irrigation/aspiration of cortical material can be performed. Extremely fine sutures may rupture during irrigation/aspiration, and some surgeons recommend an 8-0 suture such as silk, Vicryl, or Dexon; we currently use 10-0 nylon. The sutures are placed on both sides of the 12 o'clock safety suture, which is first tightened, tied, and trimmed. A suture is placed 3 mm to the right of 12 o'clock and a second 4 mm to the left (Fig. 1-32). The reason for the 3 mm spacing to the right is to permit insertion of the CooperVision Systems/Cavitron irrigation/aspiration handpiece. If an IOL is to be inserted subsequently by removing the 12 o'clock suture, a 7-mm aperture is created (i.e., 3 mm + 4 mm = 7 mm), which is wide enough to permit closed chamber insertion of most of the currently available lens implants.

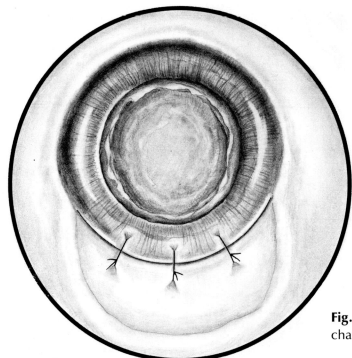

Fig. 1-32. Temporary closure of anterior chamber.

Irrigation/aspiration

The CooperVision Systems/Cavitron irrigation/aspiration handpiece is used for this. The tip aperture varies; however, the 0.3-mm aperture is the most widely used and this is what we recommend. The CooperVision Systems/Cavitron unit is set at I/A MAX, and the anterior chamber is entered in the 3-mm space between 12 o'clock and the right-hand suture. The foot pedal is depressed to position 1 (irrigation), and the aspiration port is pointed either upward or sideway. The port should always be in the surgeon's view to preclude inadvertent engagement of the posterior capsule. If the chamber deepens excessively, the irrigation bottle is too high. The CooperVision Systems/Cavitron manual should be consulted for the recommended elevation of the bottle in relation to the patient's eye. The I/A handpiece is advanced to the center of the pupil and the foot pedal is depressed to position 2 (irrigation/aspiration). The initial maneuver is to permit the aspiration to build up and let the free pieces of cortex be drawn to the tip and aspirated. This partially clears the anterior chamber of debris and permits the surgeon to assess the residual cortex, which is then aspirated in a systematic manner; to state it another way, the I/A tip is *not* moved capriciously about the anterior chamber.

It must be remembered that the residual cortex is not uniplanar; rather, it exists as a "wrapping" of the previously removed nucleus. Consider a peach with the upper third removed to expose the pit, which we liken to the nucleus. When the pit (nucleus) is removed, the residual peach (cortex) is somewhat U shaped. This approximates the situation of the residual cortex, which is as moderately adherent to the capsular cul-de-sac as the flesh of the peach is to the peach skin (Fig. 1-33). If mechanical stripping of the cortex from the capsule is added to the aspiration action of the instrument, the I/A phase of the ECCE can be expertly and expeditiously performed.

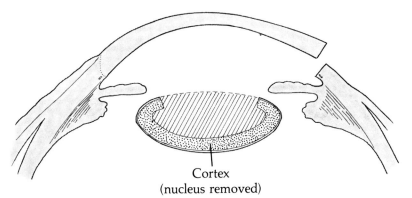

Fig. 1-33. Concept of residual cortex.

Cortex
(nucleus removed)

With this in mind our next maneuver is to engage the superior edge of residual cortex at the 3 o'clock position at the aspiration port. With continuous aspiration the tip is slowly moved back to the pupillary center, adding a stripping action to the aspiration and resulting in a large segment of cortex being aspirated (Fig. 1-34, *A*). This maneuver is continued in a clockwise direction until all cortex is aspirated (Fig. 1-34, *B* and *C*). Cortex in the superior capsular cul-de-sac can be technically difficult to remove because its presence and exposure are concealed by the iris. If this is the case, a smooth spatula or microhook held in the left hand can be inserted between the 12 o'clock and left-hand sutures to retract the iris while the superior capsular remnants are being aspirated. Elsewhere remaining pieces of cortex can be detected and removed by sliding the tip under the iris with irrigation and then activating aspiration as the tip is gently withdrawn back to the pupillary center.

If remnants of cortex remain on the posterior capsule, they should be "vacuum-cleaned" with the I/A tip set in I/A MIN (Fig. 1-34, *D*). It is important to keep the irrigating port in view; for this, a lateral oblique angulation is recommended. The tip is turned more posteriorly than in I/A MAX because mechanical debridement of posterior capsular opacities may be necessary. The *edge* of the aspiration aperture is an effective scraper especially when the aspiration is activated. It is not necessary to remove every last

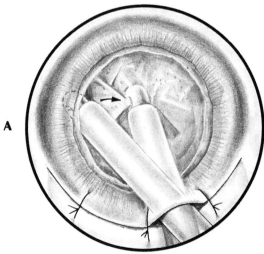

Fig. 1-34. A to **D,** Irrigation/aspiration of cortex.

STEP 1

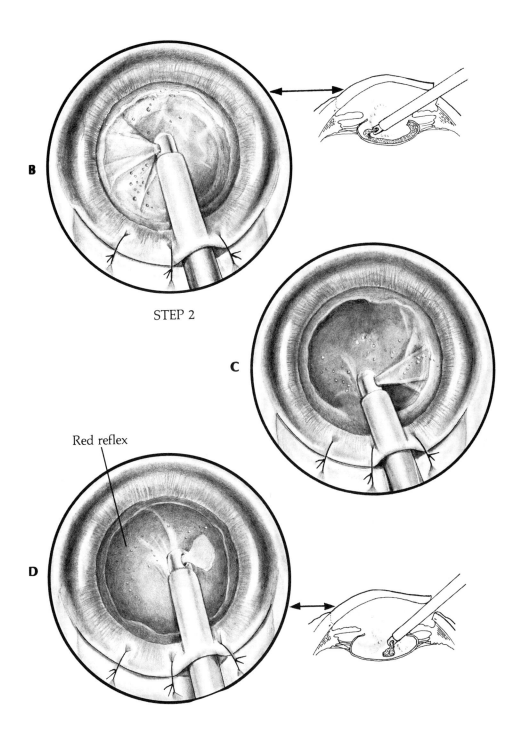

B

STEP 2

C

Red reflex

D

scrap of opacity if it will cause rupture of the posterior capsule, especially if a discission is planned. Moreover, residual capsular fibrosis may be impossible to debride, so the visual axis may have to be cleared with a discission (Fig. 1-35). The posterior capsule is to be approached with caution. When a metallic instrument is laid on the posterior capsule and is gently depressed, the coaxial microscope illumination will reflect off the metallic tip to form a halo of light 2 to 3 mm distal to the tip of the instrument. The phenomenon is more pronounced when a shiny metallic instrument is used and is seen only when the posterior capsule is intact. It is a useful test for the integrity of the posterior capsule when the surgeon is in doubt.

A peripheral iridectomy is performed by grasping the iris between the 12 o'clock and right adjacent suture (Fig. 1-36).

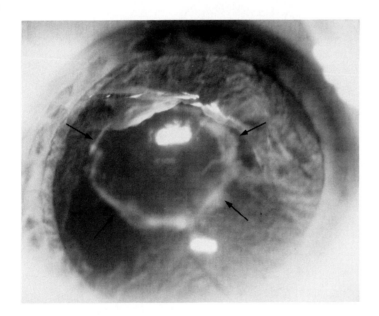

Fig. 1-35. Residual fibrosis of posterior capsule *(arrows)*.

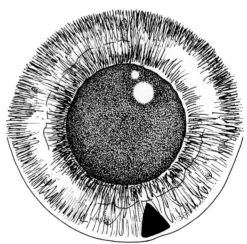

Fig. 1-36. Peripheral iridectomy (sutures not shown).

Discission

If a discission is to be performed, we advise bending a hook on a disposable 27-gauge needle as described previously (p. 23). This needle is placed on the irrigating handpiece and the CooperVision Systems/Cavitron unit is appropriately set. All air is cleared from the line and needle by irrigation. With the hook of the needle angled laterally and providing continuous irrigation, the needle is passed into the anterior chamber between the 12 o'clock and right adjacent sutures and advanced through the aperture of the peripheral iridectomy in a horizontal plane until it appears in the pupillary aperture. Be careful not to angle the discission needle posteriorly, since it may pierce the posterior capsule at the iridectomy and cause vitreous loss. The posterior capsule is engaged 2 mm inferior to the pupillary center by turning the needle point posteriorly. The posterior capsule is discissed by drawing the needle superiorly to 2 mm above the pupillary center (Fig. 1-37). Some surgeons enhance this maneuver by stopping irrigation as the needle is about to engage the posterior capsule, thus shallowing the anterior chamber and impaling the posterior capsule on the needle point. In either variation the needle is disengaged from the posterior capsule by moving it slightly inferiorly; then, after the hook is turned laterally, the needle is slowly with-

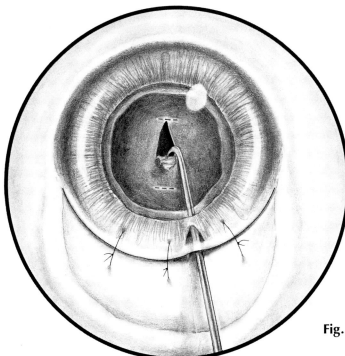

Fig. 1-37. Discission technique.

drawn from the eye. If this disengagement is not done, the capsule may still be attached to the tip of the hook, and withdrawing the hook in this position will strip the posterior capsule to the zonules at the peripheral iridectomy. The wound is closed as the surgeon prefers, using nylon sutures interspersed with the previously placed sutures (Fig. 1-38).

Comment

If an IOL is to be inserted following the ECCE, the peripheral iridectomy and discission should be performed after the implant is in situ. A debatable point is whether to prolapse the nucleus. A smaller incision can be used when the nucleus is delivered from the anterior chamber but, since complications can arise in prolapsing the nucleus (p. 40), the matter is one of surgeon preference.

A more contentious matter is whether to perform a discission. The proponents of an intact posterior capsule claim that the incidence of cystoid macular edema (CME) and retinal detachment (RD) is less in such eyes. Our own studies indicate that incidence of CME is definitely less, and our clinical experience suggests that the incidence of RD is reduced. However, if patients with an intact posterior capsule are followed long enough, 50% of the capsules will reopacify, necessitating a discission (Fig. 1-39). The advocates of discission point this out and claim that a subsequent discission is another operative procedure, not without risk, that negates the claimed advantages of an ECCE. The truth is elusive. The only advice we can give with certainty involves an ECCE or KPE in conjunction with a Shearing-type IOL (p. 142). A late discission can be technically difficult in such cases, and for this reason we perform a discission routinely at the time of the initial surgery.

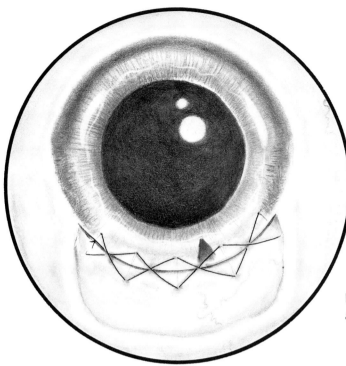

Fig. 1-38. Example of wound closure with a running suture.

Fig. 1-39. Partially opacified posterior capsule *(arrow).*

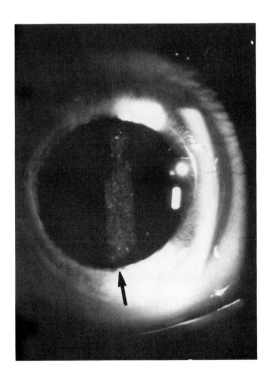

PHACOEMULSIFICATION
Incision

Correct placement of the incision is essential for the smooth execution of the phacoemulsification procedure. The incision is generally placed at the 11 o'clock position in the surgical limbus unless the physiognomy of the patient's brow or orbit precludes it. In that case the incision is made at the site where the surgeon can conveniently use the various handpieces of the CooperVision Systems/Cavitron unit. The incision should be parallel to the iris at the junction of the anterior two thirds with the posterior one third of the surgical limbus (Fig. 1-40). If the incision is too anterior, Descemet's membrane can be damaged or stripped during instrumentation. A posterior incision can be placed in eyes with deep anterior chambers, but in the average eye this may lead to iris prolapse during the procedure. The initial incision is made with a razor knife (e.g., Beaver 75L) and should be 1.5 to 2 mm, even though the incision will later to enlarged to 3 mm to accommodate the tip of the ultrasonic handpiece. An initial incision larger than 2 mm will permit excessive fluid to leak out of the eye during the anterior capsulectomy, resulting in chamber collapse with the cystotome in the eye and the possibility of corneal endothelial damage. The incision should be carefully performed with total hemostasis. All other steps in the phacoemulsification procedure are predicated on a correctly placed incision.

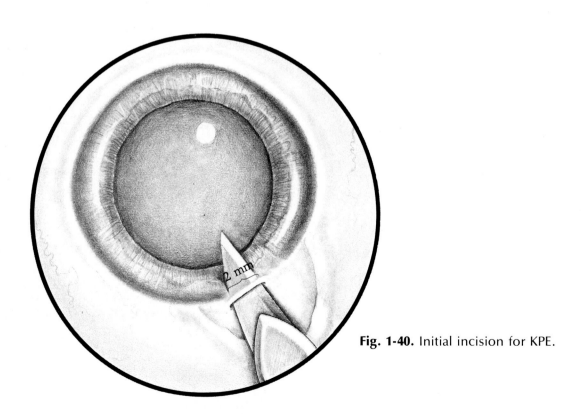

Fig. 1-40. Initial incision for KPE.

Anterior capsulectomy

This step involves the cutting of the anterior capsule of the crystalline lens, for which several techniques have been advocated. Some implant surgeons favor "tailored flaps"—deep capsular pockets into which the loops of various implants may be inserted in the expectancy of better implant fixation (p. 124). Our experience is that the phacoemulsification proceeds more easily with a large anterior capsulectomy of the can-opener variety, accomplished by using the technique already described (p. 24).

Nuclear prolapse

This is best effected with a dull irrigating cystotome because a sharp cystotome tends to slice through the nucleus as pressure is exerted. The precise technique of nuclear prolapse depends on the surgeon's preference and the hardness of the nucleus. Some surgeons precede the nuclear prolapse by loosening the nucleus from its cortical attachments by small to-and-fro movements with the cystotome (Fig. 1-41). The term *vertical seesaw* is used for the maneuver in which the cystotome engages the nucleus 2 to 3 mm inferior to

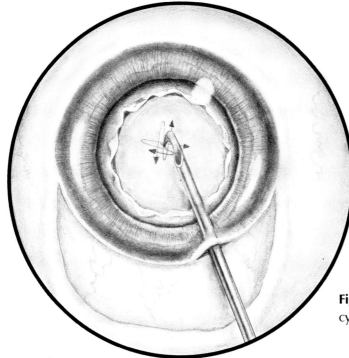

Fig. 1-41. Loosening the nucleus with cystotome. Arrows show motion.

the center of the pupil (Fig. 1-42). The cystotome, impaling the nucleus, is slowly withdrawn superiorly, pulling the inferior pole of the nucleus out of the capsular cul-de-sac and clear of the iris margin (Fig. 1-43). The nucleus is then allowed to spring inferiorly, being guided anteriorly by a "lifting" vector to the cystotome. The cystotome is released from the nucleus and repositioned in the nucleus 2 to 3 mm superior to the pupillary center. The nucleus is then moved inferiorly until the superior pole is drawn out of the superior capsular cul-de-sac and clear of the pupillary margin (Fig. 1-44), whereupon it will generally recenter anterior to the iris. A softer nucleus may require the horizontal seesaw, which is based on the same principle as the vertical seesaw but with the vectors of force exerted horizontally. Some surgeons find a combination of the vertical and horizontal maneuvers efficacious. An extremely soft nucleus cannot be prolapsed.

Prolapse of the nucleus can be difficult and can lead to complications such as vitreous loss or loss of the nucleus into the posterior chamber. A consideration of the mechanical forces involved will make nuclear prolapse easier. For example, if the surgeon pushes posteriorly too forcefully with the cystotome, the nucleus, in turn, will be pushed posteriorly and prevented from springing anteriorly over the pupillary margin. Furthermore, the horizontal axis of the nucleus is posterior to the iris plane, and a lifting vector should be added to the movements of the cystotome during nuclear prolapse. There is a knack to nuclear prolapse, which is enhanced with experience; however, the trend is toward posterior chamber phacoemulsification (p. 47).

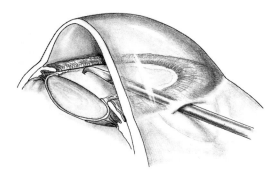

Fig. 1-42. Nucleus engaged with cystotome 2 to 3 mm inferior to center.

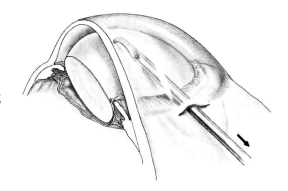

Fig. 1-43. Cystotome withdrawing, pulling inferior nuclear pole anterior to iris.

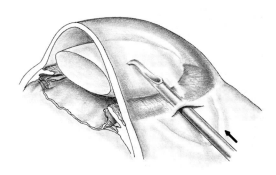

Fig. 1-44. Cystotome advancing, prolapsing superior nuclear pole anterior to iris.

EMULSIFICATION OF NUCLEUS

After the nucleus is within the anterior chamber, the initial incision is enlarged to 3 mm with a suitable blade (e.g., Beaver 55m) (Fig. 1-45). An incision smaller than this will constrict the irrigating sleeve of the ultrasonic and I/A handpieces, causing either chamber collapse or repetitive anterior chamber shallowing and deepening in positions 2 and 3. On the other hand, an incision significantly larger than 3 mm will cause chamber shallowing and frequently iris prolapse due to excessive loss of irrigating fluid around the tip of the handpieces. Attempts to deepen the anterior chamber by raising the irrigating bottle usually accelerate iris prolapse. The ultrasonic handpiece has a bevel at its tip and is inserted into the anterior chamber with the bevel orifice up, in irrigation mode. Sometimes entrance of the tip is facilitated by retracting the corneal aspect of the incision with a 0.12-mm forceps, taking care not to traumatize the irrigating sleeve. After the tip is in the eye, the machine is turned to "U/S" (ultrasonic mode) and the phacoemulsification of the nucleus begins. There are two major techniques, the "croissant" and the "carousel." The former attacks the nucleus directly at the superior pole and carves it into a U shape configuration reminiscent of a croissant (the French breakfast roll). The piece bridging the arms of the U is then phacoemulsified, breaking the nucleus into two parts (Fig. 1-46). These are attracted to the tip by the aspiration activated in foot position 2 and then emulsified with short bursts of ultrasound. Usually the power setting has to be reduced to 6 and sometimes to 4 to prevent the ultrasonic vibrations from making small pieces of nucleus careen around the anterior chamber and causing corneal endothelial trauma. In the carousel maneuver the softer periphery of the nucleus is approached first. Ultrasonic bursts shave the periphery of the nucleus as it slowly rotates (like a carousel) to the tip by the attraction of aspiration; the net result is a nucleus of much smaller diameter. If the nucleus spins too fast, the ultrasonic power should be reduced. Often the central nucleus will be too hard to emulsify completely with this technique, and whatever residue is left should be tackled directly when it is seen that the carousel maneuver is not progressing. The ultrasonic power should be turned down if the nucleus fragments ricochet off the tip during the ultrasonic mode.

As experience and confidence are gained, the ultrasonic tip will be moved around the anterior chamber less and less. The surgeon will develop a feel for how to draw the nucleus to the ultrasonic probe with aspiration. Furthermore, the surgeon should try to limit movements of the probe to a pistonlike action in the vertical plane. Lateral movements tend to be time-consuming during the ultrasonic mode and also can distort the incision. These lateral movements may pinch off the irrigating sleeve, with resultant anterior chamber collapse, or cause excess fluid loss from the anterior chamber with the same effect.

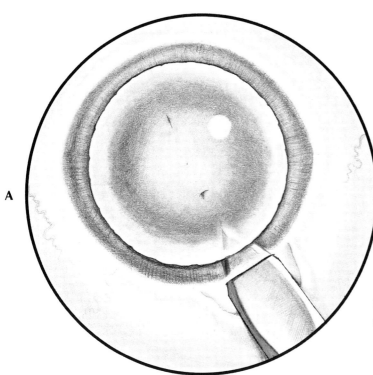

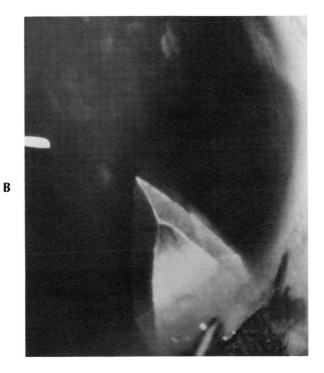

Fig. 1-45. A and **B,** Initial incision enlarged to 3 mm.

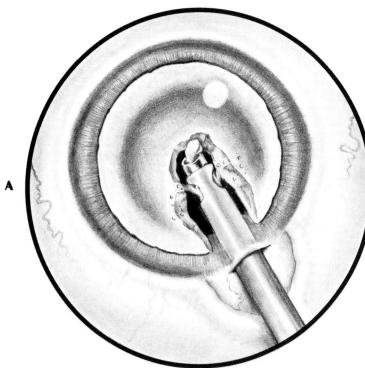

Fig. 1-46. "Croissant" technique of phacoemulsification.

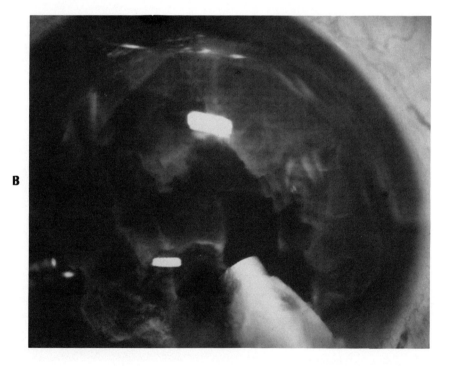

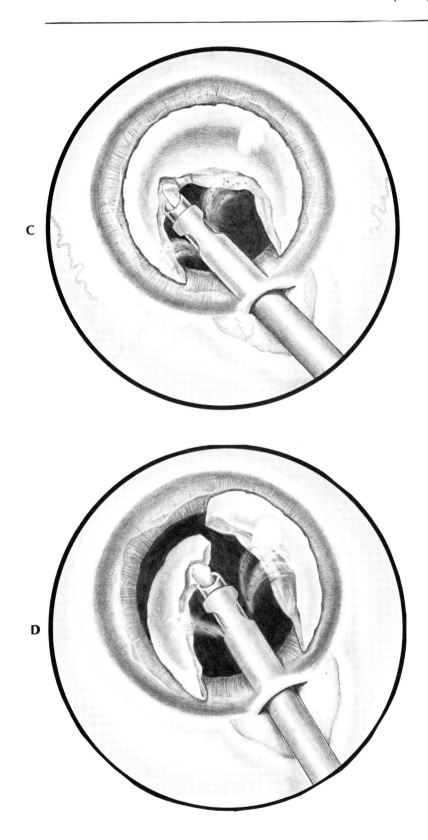

C

D

Irrigation/aspiration

The irrigation/aspiration phase is the same as for the planned ECCE already described (p. 31). Sometimes residual fragments of nucleus remain and cannot be aspirated. A second incision may be made at the 2 o'clock position, through which a fine spatula is introduced. The spatula crushes the nuclear remnant at the aspiration orifice (Fig. 1-47), i.e., "emulsifies" the nucleus, which is then aspirated. The peripheral iridectomy is now performed *unless* an implant is to be inserted, in which contingency the iridectomy is done after the implant is in situ. The technique for a peripheral iridectomy through the 3-mm phacoemulsification incision is to grab the iris through the incision with fine forceps, externalize a small knuckle of peripheral iris, and excise it. The iris is released and springs back into the anterior chamber spontaneously. Occasionally iris stroma is entrapped in the incision, whereupon it is irrigated back into the anterior chamber by a gentle jet of balanced saline solution. A discission is optional as discussed previously (p. 35). When the phacoemulsification incision is not enlarged to permit implant insertion, it can be closed with one X-shaped, horizontal mattress suture (Fig. 1-48). Our preference is 10-0 nylon, the chamber having been previously reformed with balanced saline solution.

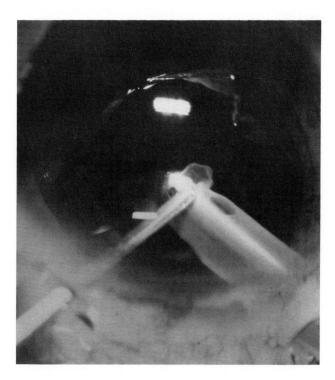

Fig. 1-47. Bimanual technique of aspirating residual nuclear fragments.

Comment

The major variation in phacoemulsification is emulsification of the nucleus in the posterior chamber, a technique preferred by many experienced surgeons. One of these expressed the opinion that the anterior chamber was the place where a beginner should work but the procedure was really best performed in the posterior chamber. The merits of this are hotly debated among ophthalmic surgeons. The case for posterior chamber phacoemulsification has several points in its favor. First, it obviates the need for initial nuclear prolapse, which can be tricky and irritating to the iris (resulting in miosis). Second, there is minimal contact with the corneal endothelium. Third, the emulsification of the nucleus is probably more efficient inasmuch as it is "held" by the nuclear cortical adhesions, which dampen any of its tendencies to move away from the probe. (They can be imagined as a gentle vise holding the nucleus for sculpting by the ultrasonic probe). Last, there are some nuclei too soft to be prolapsed; they must be emulsified in the posterior chamber.

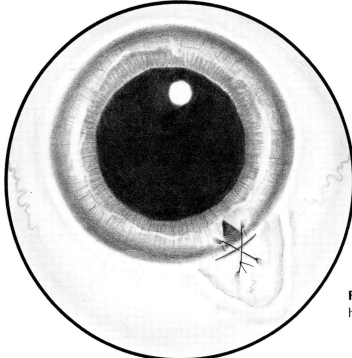

Fig. 1-48. Closure of KPE with horizontal mattress suture.

Specifically, after the anterior can opener capsulectomy, the nucleus is sculpted to a saucer shape by the ultrasonic handpiece (Fig. 1-49). At this point several options are open. Some surgeons attempt to engage the inferior aspect of the nucleus in position 2 (aspiration) and bring it forward into the anterior chamber where is is phacoemulsified. The nucleus, now much reduced in volume, is prolapsed by suction from the aspiration in this maneuver. Other surgeons use a two-instrument technique by introducing a

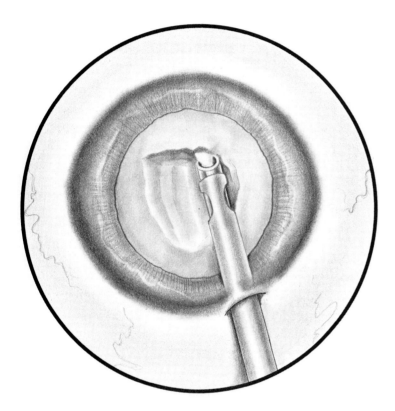

Fig. 1-49. Nucleus saucerized with ultrasound.

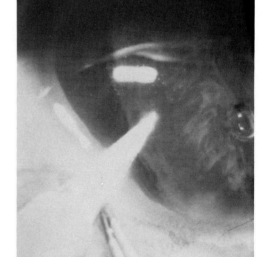

Fig. 1-50. Second incision at 2 o'clock position at surgical limbus.

fine spatula or nucleus rotator into the anterior chamber with the left hand through either the initial incision or (our preference) a second stab incision at 2 to 3 o'clock in the surgical limbus (Fig. 1-50). With this second instrument the inferior pole of the nucleus is moved inferoposteriorly, thus presenting the superior pole to the phacoemulsification tip (Fig. 1-51), which nibbles away the residual nucleus (Fig. 1-52) in the ultrasonic mode. The sculpting of the nucleus produces a vertical ridge at the inferior third of nucleus, and

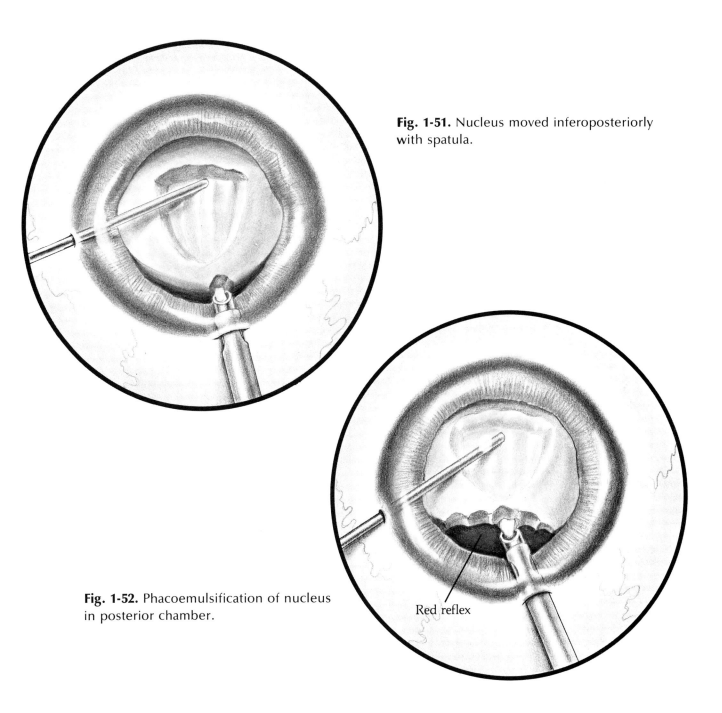

Fig. 1-51. Nucleus moved inferoposteriorly with spatula.

Fig. 1-52. Phacoemulsification of nucleus in posterior chamber.

Red reflex

the left-hand instrument is placed against this ridge (Fig. 1-53, *A*). As the inferior pole of the nucleus is moved inferoposteriorly, the foot-switch is placed in position 0 (no irrigation). The anterior chamber slowly shallows and, as the contents of the posterior chamber move forward, the superior pole of the nucleus is pushed anteriorly, where it is secured with the tip of the ultrasonic handpiece and braced. The footswitch is then depressed to position 1 (irrigation), which deepens the anterior chamber, pushing the posterior capsule posteriorly, and leaves the superior pole of the nucleus anteriorly, against the ultrasonic tip (Fig. 1-53, *B*). The left-hand instrument is repositioned against the left lateral edge of the nucleus. By slowly rotating successive areas of the nucleus counterclockwise to the ultrasonic tip, it is emulsified.

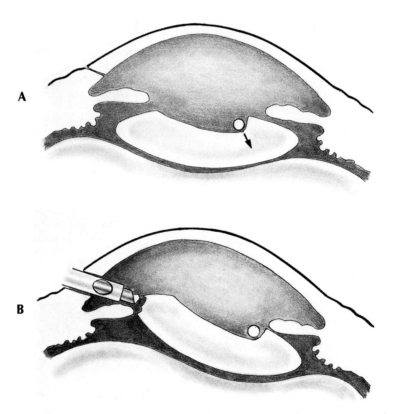

Fig. 1-53. A and **B,** Schematic of bimanual posterior chamber phacoemulsification.

Yet another alternative is to withdraw the ultrasonic probe, turn the machine to "standby," and insert the irrigating cystotome. Assuming the pupil has remained adequately dilated, the sculpted (hence smaller) nucleus may now be prolapsed with the seesaw maneuvers, aided by a second-instrument approach if necessary. The phacoemulsification is then completed in the anterior chamber. The subsequent steps are as described previously. The disadvantage of posterior chamber phacoemulsification is the danger of violating the posterior capsule and/or losing vitreous with possible subluxation of nuclear material into the posterior chamber. The arena for phacoemulsification is bounded anteriorly by the corneal endothelium and posteriorly by the posterior capsule; anterior chamber phacoemulsification avoids the latter and posterior chamber phacoemulsification avoids the former. Ultimately the surgeon's own experience will serve as guide.

Two

Anterior chamber intraocular lenses

GENERAL PRINCIPLES

The first anterior chamber lens implant, using the angle for support, was inserted by Baron of France in 1952. Strampelli followed in 1953 with an angle-supported lens of his own design, which he reported at the congress of the Societas Lombardos di Oftalmologica in Pavia, Italy, a few months later. Numerous surgeons designed, thereafter, their own versions of anterior chamber lenses, but disaster was to lay ahead in the form of late corneal decompensation.

Notwithstanding setbacks and in spite of formidable obstacles and professional criticism, Choyce of England persisted. His perseverance established the feasibility of anterior chamber fixation and produced by evolution an anterior chamber, angle-fixated intraocular lens that has stood the test of time (Fig. 2-1). Choyce's name is synonymous with anterior chamber lens implants; in recognition of this, he was awarded the American Intra-Ocular Implant Society's Binkhorst Medal in 1981.

Other lens implants of this type have now appeared and are discussed in this chapter; but let us consider the advantages of anterior chamber fixation. First, the lens may be inserted after an ECCE, ICCE, or KPE. Second, iris sutures are not required for IOL fixation, and iris retraction is not necessary for IOL insertion. The single-plane design permits insertion without corneal retraction and preserves a formed anterior chamber. Last, the pupil may be dilated postoperatively ad lib. (Fig. 2-2) without fear of IOL dislocation, and iris defects (e.g., surgical coloboma) may be "bridged" by the IOL without iris suturing (p. 212).

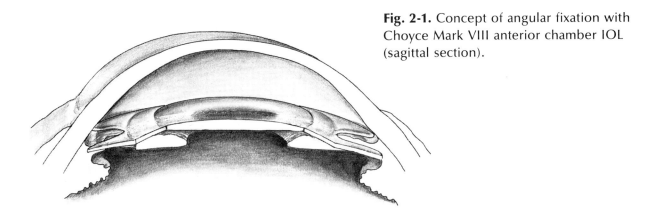

Fig. 2-1. Concept of angular fixation with Choyce Mark VIII anterior chamber IOL (sagittal section).

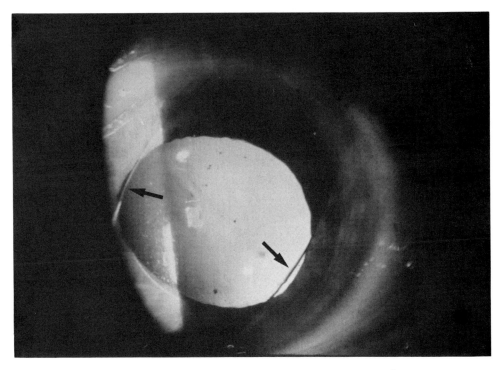

Fig. 2-2. Pupillary dilatation with Choyce Mark VIII. Note pupillary margin beyond edge of IOL *(arrows)*.

All currently available anterior chamber IOLs have two significant disadvantages. First, obstructions of the angle such as peripheral anterior synechiae may preclude insertion of this type of implant or at least dictate a change in the axis of insertion. Therefore gonioscopy is an important part of the preoperative examination (Fig. 2-3). Second, the IOL *length* has to be considered prior to implantation in a given eye. Obviously, patients' anterior chamber dimensions will vary, and if a lens is excessively short, it will rotate in the anterior chamber (Chapter 8). Conversely, if it is too long, excessive pressure will be exerted at the angle. For this reason, anterior chamber lenses are supplied in a variety of lengths, generally 11.0 to 13.5 mm, in 0.5-mm increments. A surgeon or hospital therefore requires an enlarged inventory because different lengths as well as dioptric powers must be stocked.

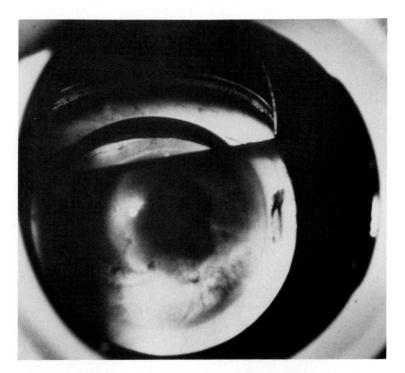

Fig. 2-3. Preoperative gonioscopy (Courtesy Dr. D. Peter Choyce.)

How is the correct length for a given patient ascertained? Choyce advocates measuring the horizontal corneal diameter, limbal white to limbal white, with calipers (Fig. 2-4). To this measurement 1.0 mm is added to give the correct IOL length regardless of the axis of insertion. This method has been questioned by Heslin, who recommends using a calibrated "dipstick" designed by Kelman to verify the internal diameter of the anterior chamber intraoperatively. In our experience, Choyce's rule is correct most of the time. The management of exceptions is discussed later.

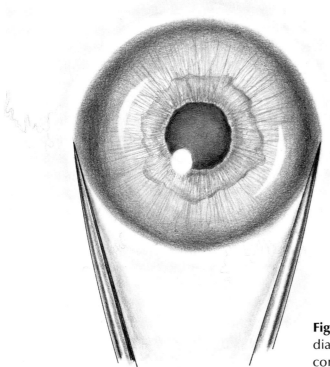

Fig. 2-4. Calipers measuring corneal diameter "white to white" to ascertain correct IOL length.

Choyce anterior chamber IOLs

Choyce modified Strampelli's original lens in a series of successive steps culminating in the Choyce Mark VIII, designed by him in 1963. In the evolution of the Choyce Mark VIII IOL, the haptic portion's thickness was markedly reduced from that of the Strampelli lens. Furthermore, Choyce's lens is quadripedal, whereas the Strampelli lens had a tripod design.

Description. In Fig. 2-5, it should be noted that the length of a Choyce lens is determined by the *diagonal* length between opposite foot tips, i.e., the length is the diameter of the circle centered at the optical center of the

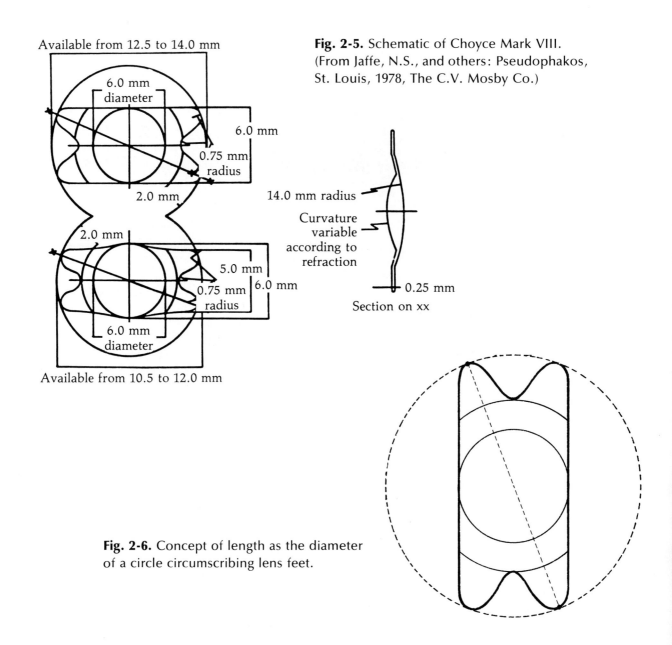

Fig. 2-5. Schematic of Choyce Mark VIII. (From Jaffe, N.S., and others: Pseudophakos, St. Louis, 1978, The C.V. Mosby Co.)

Available from 12.5 to 14.0 mm

6.0 mm diameter

6.0 mm

0.75 mm radius

2.0 mm

2.0 mm

5.0 mm

0.75 mm radius

6.0 mm

6.0 mm diameter

Available from 10.5 to 12.0 mm

14.0 mm radius

Curvature variable according to refraction

0.25 mm

Section on xx

Fig. 2-6. Concept of length as the diameter of a circle circumscribing lens feet.

implant, whose inscription just touches the tips of each of the four IOL feet (Fig. 2-6). It should also be observed that the original Choyce Mark VIII is rhomboidal in lengths of 12.0 mm and less (Fig. 2-7). In lengths of 12.5 mm and greater the IOL is rectangular (Fig. 2-8). The Choyce lens has a biconvex optic (Fig. 2-9, *A*). Tennant modified the Choyce Mark VIII by making the optic planoconvex with the convex surface anterior (Fig. 2-9, *B*), but in all other aspects the Tennant lens closely parallels the Choyce Mark VIII.

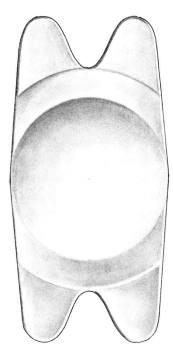

Fig. 2-7. Rhomboidal Choyce Mark VIII, lengths 12.00 mm and less.

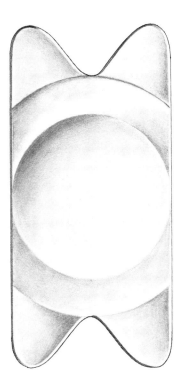

Fig. 2-8. Rectangular Choyce Mark VIII, lengths 12.5 mm and longer.

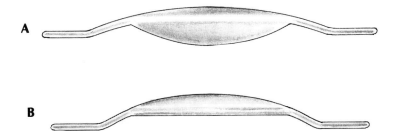

Fig. 2-9. A, Biconvex Choyce optic. **B,** Planoconvex Tennant optic.

Operation. Some controversy exists about whether the IOL should be inserted horizontally or vertically (Fig. 2-10). A horizontal insertion is suggested by Choyce, but this can be awkward for a microsurgeon accustomed to working from a superior exposure. Tennant inserts his lens in a vertical axis, but this also has its drawbacks in a patient with a prominent brow or deep-set orbit. In these patients the advancing feet can be angulated excessively posteriorly and "snow ploughed" into the iris and possibly into the anterior hyaloid face. For this reason we insert the Choyce Mark VIII obliquely (Fig. 2-11, *A*), from a superior temporal incision, but no consensus exists and we cannot be dogmatic on this point.

In single-plane pseudophakia our rule for the minimal incision size for IOL insertion is the optic plus 1.0 mm. Since the Choyce Mark VIII has a 6.0-mm optic, 7.0 mm would be the minimum size for incision. In the case of an ICCE or ECCE, the incision is closed down to 7.0 mm. A KPE requires that the section be enlarged to 7.0 mm. The insertion should be performed under air bubble, but the iris should be horizontal *not* concave. The latter predisposes to "tucking" of the iris, as the inferior feet advance across the anterior chamber. *Iris tuck* is discussed later in this chapter.

The right foot of the implant is grasped (Fig. 2-11, *B*) with Clayman for-

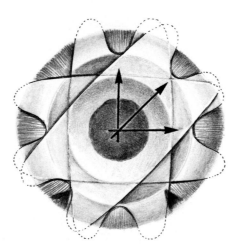

Fig. 2-10. Possible variation in axis of insertion of Choyce IOL.

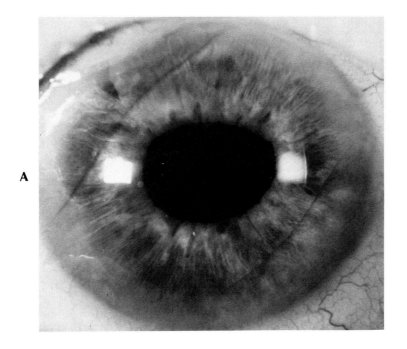

A

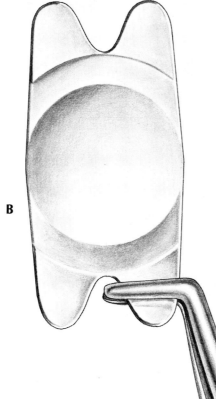

B

Fig. 2-11. **A,** Choyce Mark VIII inserted obliquely.
B, Right foot of IOL grasped with forceps.

ceps, and the IOL is introduced through the incision and slid across the anterior chamber until the distal feet rest in the inferior angle (Fig. 2-12). The forceps are released, leaving the two proximal (superior) feet protruding from the section. The scleral lip is grasped between the two feet by fine-toothed forceps held in the left hand. Clayman forceps, held in the right, are turned so that the tips point posteriorly. As the sclera is retracted up and out, the right foot of the IOL is tapped into position (Fig. 2-13). The sclera is then regrasped to the left of the left foot, and that foot is similarly tapped into position. This type of IOL centers well spontaneously without much additional intracameral manipulation.

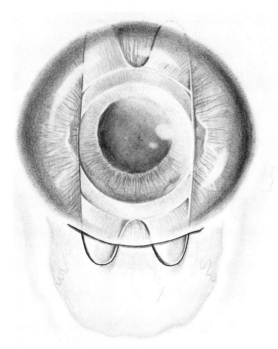

Fig. 2-12. Distal feet in inferior angle.

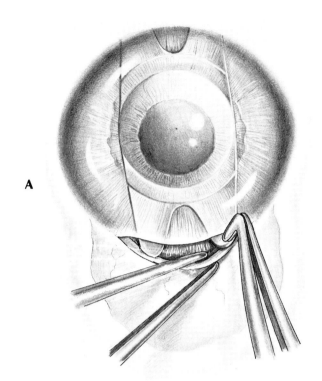

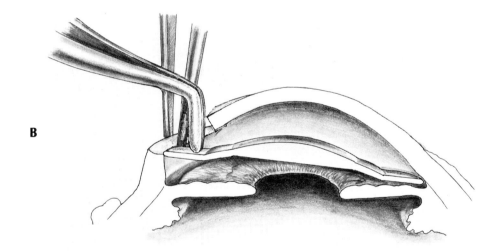

Fig. 2-13. A, Right proximal foot tapped into position. **B,** Sagittal view of positioning proximal feet.

The peripheral iridectomies are critically important (Fig. 2-14), first because there may be a higher incidence of pupillary block in this type of IOL (Chapter 7), and second because the iridectomies serve as markers, by which intracameral postoperative IOL rotation if any, can be ascertained by observing the relationship of the foot plates to the iridectomies (Fig. 8-4). We perform an iridectomy on each side of the superior feet and an optional iridectomy between the two superior feet as may be required to prevent internal iris prolapse. The lateral iridectomies should not be immediately adjacent to the superior feet, lest one of the feet prolapse through an iridectomy following postoperative rotation. After the iridectomies are placed and the anterior chamber reformed, there still may be internal iris prolapse. This refers to an area of iris bowing anteriorly around the IOL, presumably caused by misdirected aqueous flow. It must be rectified; a midstromal iridotomy is performed with fine scissors in the area of internal iris prolapse (Fig. 2-15), if the prolapse persists and does not flatten with reformation of the anterior chamber (Fig. 2-16).

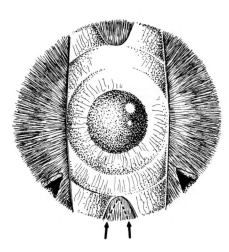

Fig. 2-14. Usual position of peripheral iridectomies with Choyce Mark VIII. Broken line *(arrows)* shows optional site for a third peripheral iridectomy between two proximal feet.

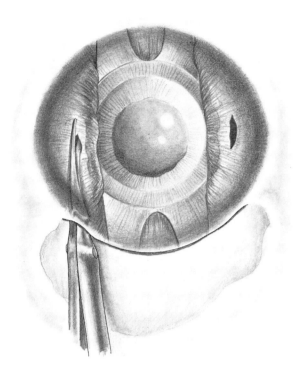

Fig. 2-15. Midstromal iridotomies to relieve internal iris prolapse.

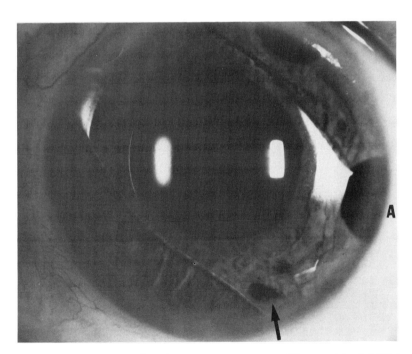

Fig. 2-16. Midstromal iridotomy *(arrow)* in a Choyce Mark VIII inserted. Parenthetically, IOL has rotated posoperatively. Note foot in peripheral iridectomy *(A)* and occlusion of midstromal iridotomy by IOL body.

Is the IOL the correct size for the eye? If the IOL's superior feet simply fall into position, the IOL is probably too short. On the other hand, if excessive retraction of the scleral lip is required to position the superior feet, the IOL is too long. Choyce states that if more than 1.5 mm of the superior feet protrude through the section when the distal feet are in situ, the IOL is too long; but this rule surely depends on how far posteriorly the incision has been made and has not been very useful in our experience. Tennant devised the "nudge" test and the "tap" test. In the former an instrument is inserted into the inverted V between the two superior feet after the IOL is in situ. Gentle inferior movement of the IOL should *not* bring the superior feet into view, unless the IOL is too short. The tap test is performed after the incision is closed and the anterior chamber reformed. The sclera is gently depressed over the pars plana 90 degrees to the long axis of the IOL. The iris should move but *not* the IOL, unless it is too short (Fig. 2-17). With experience none of these tests are necessary. The surgeon develops a feel for the correctness of the fit as the lens is inserted. Any IOL that does not have the correct fit should be exchanged at surgery to prevent postoperative complications. In the case of a short IOL, there would be recurrent iritis and possible corneal

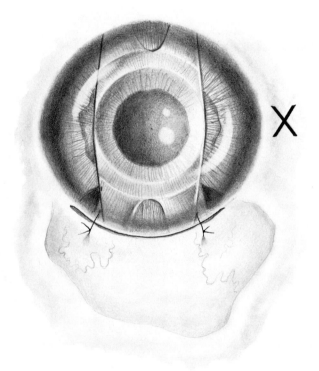

Fig. 2-17. Tap test. Sclera is gently depressed at *X.* Iris should move but not IOL if it is the correct length.

edema from a mobile intraocular foreign body (i.e., the IOL). When the IOL is too long, it often settles posteriorly at an increased chord length within the anterior chamber. In this position it invaginates the iris and pushes it against the ciliary body. The result can be recurrent iritis and ocular tenderness. Marked astigmatism can also be produced from an overly long IOL.

Even eyes with the correct length Choyce Mark VIII and Tennant IOLs exhibit ocular tenderness for many months postoperatively. Consideration of this and concern about pupillary block hastened the trend to a new generation of anterior chamber lens characterized by less area of polymethylmethacrylate within the eye, i.e., less IOL bulk. Choyce designed the Mark IX model, which is available with 4.0-mm (Fig. 2-18, *A*) and 5.0-mm optics (Fig. 2-18, *B*). Compare the area to a Mark VIII (Fig. 2-18, *C*). The method of

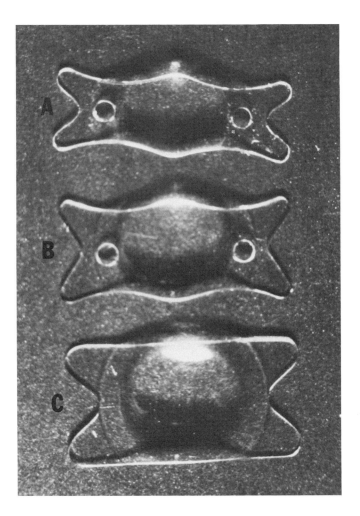

Fig. 2-18. A, Choyce Mark IX 4-mm optic. **B,** Choyce Mark IX 5-mm optic. **C,** Choyce Mark VIII 6-mm optic. (Courtesy Dr. D. Peter Choyce.)

insertion is identical to the technique described previously, and the 5.0-mm optic model seems to be a further viable evolutionary step (Fig. 2-19). We consider a 4.0-mm optic too small: in dim illumination the pupil will dilate and the patient will have simultaneous aphakic and pseudophakic vision.

Comments. The Choyce Mark VIII exemplifies one of the great advantages of most anterior chamber IOLs: the IOL's independence from iris and pupil integrity except in the most extreme cases. Fig. 2-20 shows an anterior chamber lens inserted in an eye with multiple sphincter ruptures. An iris-fixated IOL would have been contraindicated here. Moreover, an anterior chamber lens can be inserted, "bridging" a sector iridectomy (Fig. 2-21) and obviating the need for additional iris surgery as described in Chapter 7.

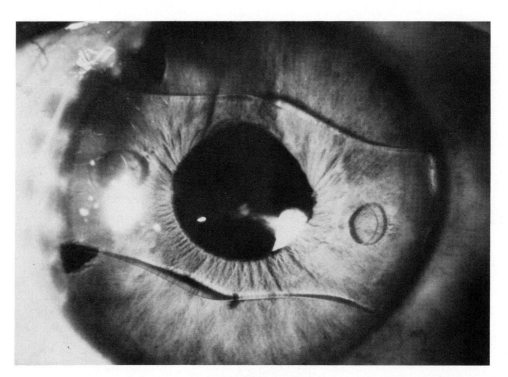

Fig. 2-19. Horizontal placement of Choyce Mark IX with 5-mm optic. (Courtesy Dr. D. Peter Choyce.)

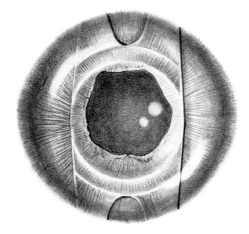

Fig. 2-20. Choyce Mark VIII in eye with multiple sphincter ruptures.

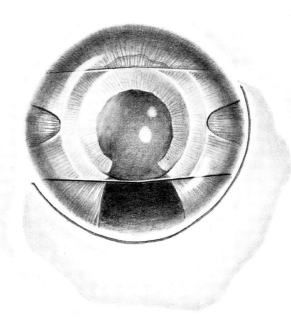

Fig. 2-21. Choyce Mark VIII inserted horizontally to bridge a sector iridectomy.

Kelman anterior chamber IOLs

Kelman has designed a lens that appears as an inverted 7 (Fig. 2-22). This lens fixates at three points intracamerally and is of markedly reduced surface area in comparison with the Choyce Mark VIII. The Kelman lens's three-point fixation (Fig. 2-23) differs from the original tripod concept of Strampelli in that its feet form angles not to each other but to a broad-based triangle—analogous to the three legs of a dairymaid's stool.

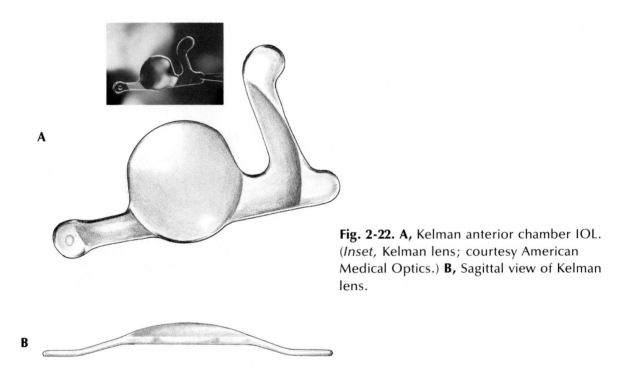

Fig. 2-22. A, Kelman anterior chamber IOL. (*Inset,* Kelman lens; courtesy American Medical Optics.) **B,** Sagittal view of Kelman lens.

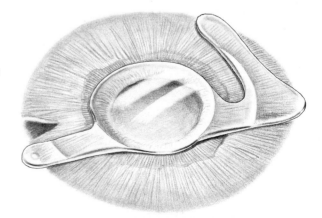

Fig. 2-23. Concept of three-point fixation of Kelman lens.

Description. The Kelman lens has an optic approximately 5.5 mm in diameter and therefore is amenable to small incision surgery. A KPE would be enlarged to a 6.5-mm section, and an ICCE or ECCE would be closed, leaving a 6.5-mm section.

Operation. To insert the Kelman lens, the optic should be grasped near the junction with the superior foot. The anterior chamber should be formed and, if air is used, care should be taken not to make the iris diaphragm excessively concave for the reasons noted previously. In Fig. 2-24 the toe of the inferior foot *(A)* is slid through the incision with a motion to the surgeon's left. The motion is continued until the heel *(B)* can be pivoted into the anterior chamber (Fig. 2-25). There is a knack to this crucial part of the insertion, which is facilitated by momentarily weakening the forceps' grip on the optic and then regrasping it, when the surgeon's hand and forceps are in a comfortable position to rotate the heel into the anterior chamber.

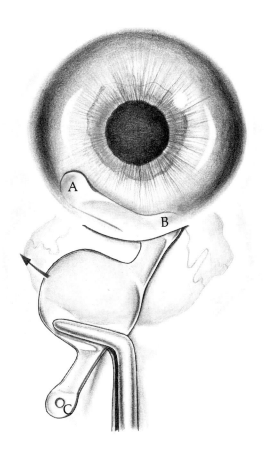

Fig. 2-24. Toe *(A)* of Kelman IOL inserted into anterior chamber with a motion to surgeon's left. *B,* Heel; *C,* superior foot.

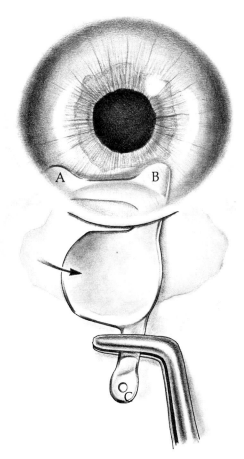

Fig. 2-25. IOL is pivoted so that heel *(B)* passes into anterior chamber.

When this is accomplished, the IOL is advanced across the anterior chamber (Fig. 2-26) until the implant forceps come in contact with the incision. The implant forceps are loosened and slid up the superior foot of the implant to regrasp the superior tip and slide the lens further across the anterior chamber, until the inferior foot (*A* and *B*) are in the inferior angle. The implant forceps are released. The superior foot *(C)* is positioned by retracting the scleral aspect of the incision up and out and tapping the superior foot into the anterior chamber (Fig. 2-27), where it comes to rest in the superior angle.

The peripheral iridectomy should be superior but as far away from the superior foot as the limits of the incision will allow (Fig. 2-28). The reason for this is that if the superior foot were to rotate and prolapse posteriorly through the peripheral iridectomy, the whole lens would be destabilized because triangular fixation is lost when the apex of the triangle is no longer fixated. This is a potential problem for this type of implant and is discussed in Chapter 8. Lenses that have quadripedal fixation, such as the Choyce Mark IX, are less likely to destabilize but on the other hand are more rigid. It seems that the Kelman lens has some degree of flexibility and will be more forgiving if it is slightly too long.

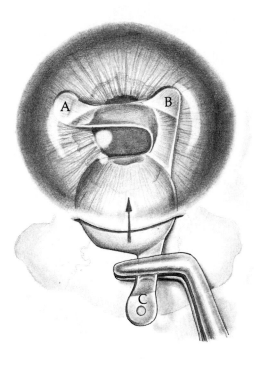

Fig. 2-26. IOL is slid across anterior chamber to inferior angle.

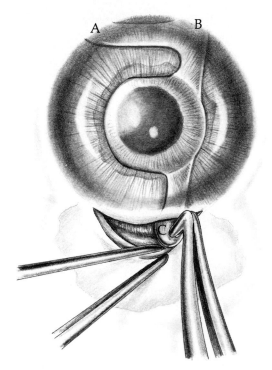

Fig. 2-27. Superior foot *(C)* is tapped into position.

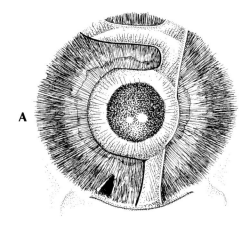

Fig. 2-28. **A,** Kelman lens in situ; note position of peripheral iridectomy. **B,** Kelman lens in situ, peripheral iridectomy too close to superior foot.

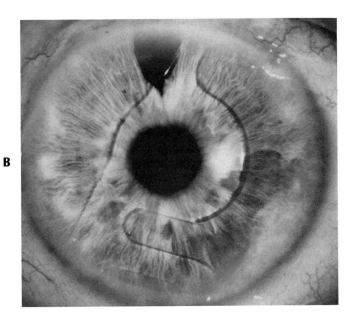

After the Kelman lens is inserted, the section is closed and a discission is performed, if the operative technique dictates. The lens position can be somewhat adjusted with a smooth spatula, but once in situ a correctly sized lens moves very little. The surgeon should be careful that the free edge of the optic is not tilted posteriorly. We have seen cases in which this edge has been "captured" by the constricting pupil. Another theoretical problem is the anatomic position of the pupil, which when constricted, is not in the center of the anterior chamber but slightly nasal. Considering the variations in patient population it is conceivable that some pupils may coincide with the periphery of the Kelman lens, and that differences may exist between the right and left eyes. However, this lens generally centers very well (Fig. 2-29).

Other lenses

Other contemporary anterior chamber lenses are available, such as the Tennant anchor lens (Fig. 2-30) and the Kelman Quadraflex (Figs. 2-31 and 2-32), and surely other inventors are currently working on innovative designs. The principles of insertion remain the same.

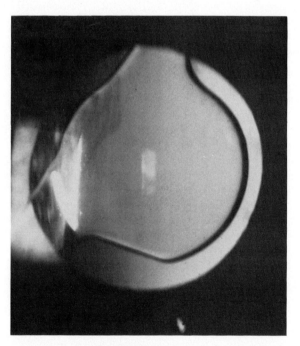

Fig. 2-29. Excellent centration of Kelman IOL shown in patient with dilated pupil.

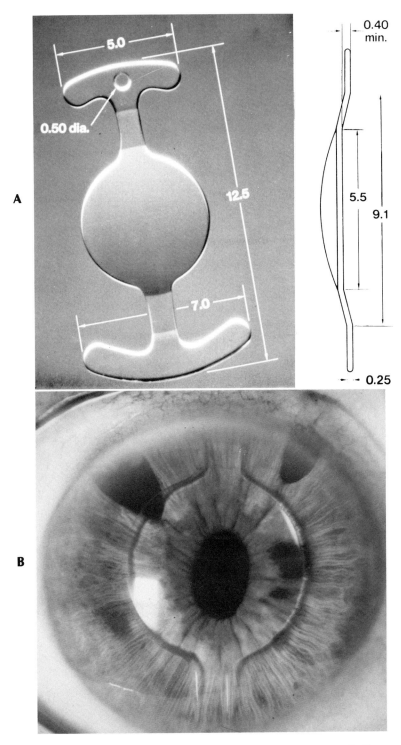

Fig. 2-30. A, Tennant anchor lens. (Courtesy Precision-Cosmet.) **B,** Tennant anchor lens in situ. Note pupil is slightly oval, presumably secondary to minimal surgeon-induced iris tuck (p. 80).

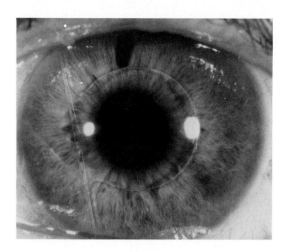

Fig. 2-31. Kelman Quadraflex IOL in situ. (Courtesy Dr. C. Kelman.)

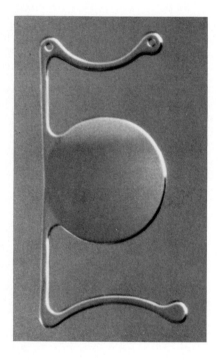

Fig. 2-32. Kelman Quadraflex anterior chamber IOL. (Courtesy Cilco, Inc.)

There is also a trend toward flexible anterior chamber lenses as exemplified by the Leiske lens (Fig. 2-33). In this lens the optic is solid polymethylmethacrylate (PMMA), but the loops are flexible PMMA. The current flexible anterior chamber lenses may seem a recidivist step to students of intraocular lens history, inasmuch as they have a resemblance to a similar lens designed and abandoned by Dannheim many years ago. The problem with the Dannheim lens was degradation of the loops, which were made of nylon (Supramid). The current designs obviate this risk by using PMMA, a plastic that has proved inert within the eye. In our combined experience we have never seen nor heard of intraocular degradation of PMMA.

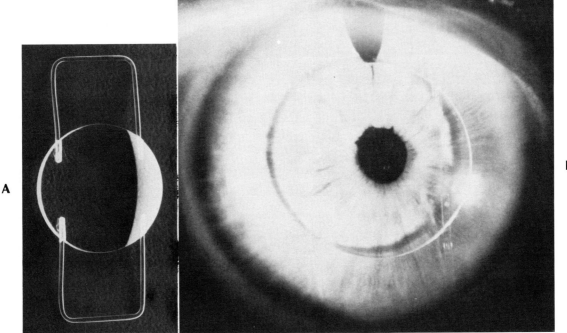

Fig. 2-33. A, Leiske anterior chamber IOL. **B,** Leiske anterior chamber IOL in situ. (**A** courtesy Surgidev Corp. and Dr. Larry Leiske; **B** courtesy Dr. Larry Leiske.)

Hessberg has designed a flexible-looped anterior chamber lens in which the loops are fabricated from polypropylene (Fig. 2-34). Azar devised a polypropylene lens but with a different loop configuration (Fig. 2-35). Investigations in Japan and Europe have suggested that polypropylene is susceptible to ultraviolet degradation, but at wavelengths deflected by the cornea. On the basis of current knowledge polypropylene is a viable loop material for anterior chamber lenses.

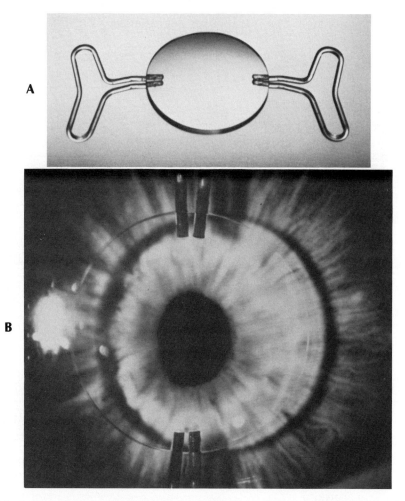

Fig. 2-34. A, Hessberg anterior chamber IOL. **B,** Hessberg anterior chamber IOL in situ. (Courtesy Intermedics Intraocular.)

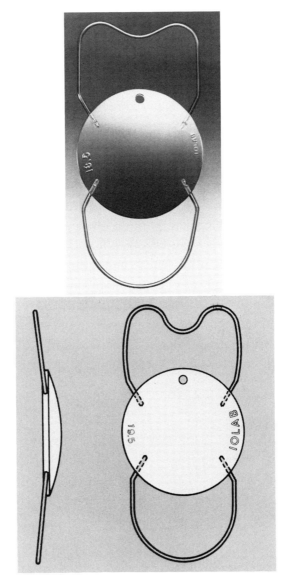

Fig. 2-35. Azar anterior chamber lens.
(Courtesy, Iolab Corp.)

Comments. An interesting question is whether a flexible anterior chamber lens implant can accommodate a range of lens lengths and thus obviate the need of an enlarged inventory and complications related to missized lenses. An anterior chamber lens that is too shoi. will be a loose foreign body within the eye, irrespective of whether it is rigid or flexible. But what about a longer flexible lens? For example, could a 13.0-mm flexible lens be suitable for eyes requiring lenses ranging from 12.5 to 13.0 mm? This range encompasses most adult eyes, and a single lens size would be advantageous to the ophthalmologic profession.

The advantages of such a lens must be weighed against the disadvantages. First, the spring action of the flexible loops and the resultant pressure in the angle of some eyes may be deleterious. Second, when an anterior chamber lens is inserted in an eye whose anterior chamber requires a shorter length, the only way the lens can accommodate to the anterior chamber is to reduce its length by bowing anteriorly. This could put the optic excessively close to the corneal endothelium. Hyperopic eyes often have shallower anterior chambers and require IOLs of higher dioptric powers and hence thicker optics. Therefore these eyes could be in double jeopardy. Notwithstanding, a universal anterior chamber lens would be desirable; Shepard has devised an anterior chamber IOL that may have this feature (Fig. 2-36).

Finally, anterior chamber lenses lend themselves well to secondary lens implantation, which is the insertion of a lens implant at a time remote from the initial cataract surgery. This important topic is discussed in Chapter 10.

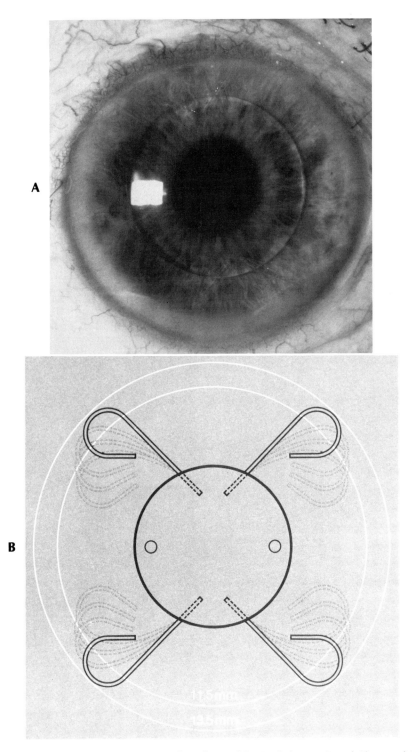

Fig. 2-36. A, Shepard anterior chamber IOL. **B,** Schematic of Shepard IOL. Note that lens is designed to accommodate lengths of 11.5 to 13.5 mm. (**A** courtesy Dr. Dennis Shepard; **B** courtesy Surgidev Corp.)

Iris tuck

Iris tuck refers to the entrapment of peripheral iris tissue in the angle by the feet or loops of an anterior chamber lens, and it occurs as the lens is slid across the anterior chamber. If the advancing portion of the IOL is angled too posteriorly, it will push iris ahead of it, trapping it in the angle. A fold (or tuck) of iris will then be permanently installed between the distal feet or loop of the IOL and the adjacent angle. The tuck cannot be alleviated once the IOL is in situ; if noted during surgery, the IOL should be partially withdrawn and reinserted correctly. An oval pupil with the vertical axis corresponding to the vertical axis of the IOL is pathognomonic of iris tuck but may be so subtle as to pass unnoticed during the operation (see Fig. 2-30, *B*). Postoperatively, it is readily observed during a slit lamp examination, and the degree of pupillary ovalling may increase as the postoperative time lengthens.

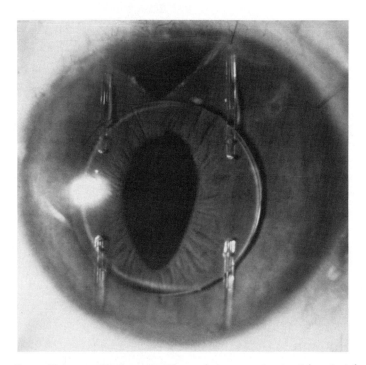

Fig. 2-37. Pupil ovalling, secondary to iris tuck in a patient with a Leiske anterior chamber IOL.

Iris tuck is surgeon induced and may be avoided with careful technique. Its principal cause is insertion of the IOL into an eye with a concave iris, which tends to tuck the iris. The iris should be horizontal for optimum anterior chamber IOL insertion. A second cause of iris tuck is an excessively long anterior chamber IOL. If the lens is too long, it will have to occupy a longer chord length within the eye—hence a more posterior position than a correctly sized lens. The result is frequently iris tuck, chronic ocular tenderness, and excessive astigmatism based on distortion of the globe. Other complications of an excessively long IOL are discussed on p. 228.

A moderate degree of iris tuck (Fig. 2-30, *B*) is of no significance, except perhaps cosmetic. Excessive iris tuck (Fig. 2-37) is usually accompanied by pain and a chronic ocular inflammatory syndrome, of which CME is often a part. The treatment in these cases is implant removal, which is discussed on p. 273.

Three

Iris-fixation intraocular lenses

GENERAL PRINCIPLES

All of the iris-fixation lens implants are held in position, as their name would imply, by the iris and are designed so that their optic portion coincides with the pupil. Because pupil size varies with light and accommodation, these lenses must be adequately fixated to prevent dislocation. The lens styles currently in use are a result of evolution, particularly in overall loop diameter. There are some subtle differences between manufacturers that may modify the position of the iris-fixation sutures and the length of the suture bite. For this reason the surgeon should be thoroughly familiar with the lens being used.

BINKHORST STYLE IRIS CLIP LENS IMPLANT (4-LOOP CLIP LENS)

This implant may be used after either an intracapsular, extracapsular, or phacoemulsification procedure. It is also suitable for some secondary intraocular lens implantations (p. 283). The implant can be compared to a paper clip, and the iris to the paper in the clip. However, the iris is not grabbed by the loops but rather should slide between them (Fig. 3-1). The spacing between the anterior and posterior loops is ideally 0.5 to 0.6 mm. Anything less than this makes insertion difficult, and more space causes the lens to ride too anteriorly (with danger of corneal touch) and also produces excessive pseudophacodonesis.

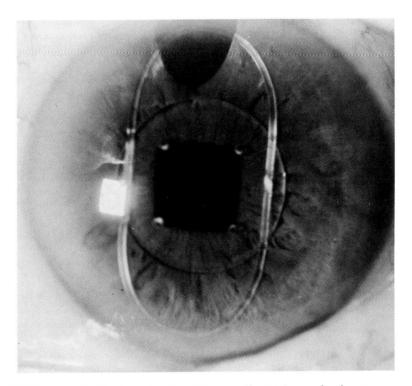

Fig. 3-1. Binkhorst iris clip lens in situ. (From Jaffe, N.S., and others: Pseudophakos, St. Louis, 1978, The C.V. Mosby Co.)

Description

The lens has a 5.0-mm diameter optic, occupying a prepupillary position in situ. Most manufacturers use a planoconvex configuration for the optic with the convex surface anterior; however, there is available a model with a biconvex optic. There are two pairs of loops, anterior and posterior, the anterior and posterior designation referring to the loops' position in situ relative to the iris. Polypropylene is the polymer currently used by most U.S. manufacturers as loop material, but nylon-6 (Supramid) is preferred by some European companies. Overall diameter of the anterior loops should be 7.5 to 8.0 mm and 8.5 to 9.0 mm for the posterior loops. The space between the loops should be 0.5 to 0.6 mm for the reasons already given. The posterior angulation of about 10 degrees in both pairs of loops was an important evolutionary step in the design of this lens and is most desirable (Fig. 3-2). It keeps the apexes of the anterior loops clear of the endothelium and also conforms to the configuration of the iris and the anterior hyaloid face. On the other hand, if the angulation is excessive, it will bow the optic forward with the danger of corneal endothelial touch and pseudophacodonesis.

Operation

A 5.0-mm pupil size after cataract extraction is desirable for ease of insertion. For pupils larger than this, intracameral acetylcholine may be instilled. A miotic pupil will require iris retraction with the surgeon's left hand, and extreme miosis can necessitate an iridoplasty (Chapter 7).

To insert the implant, the optic should be grasped with Clayman forceps (Fig. 3-3). The optic is held where the right arm of the anterior superior loop emanates from the optic. The surgeon should beware of "tiddlywinking," whereby the optic springs out of the jaws of the forceps as they are being closed. It is important *not* to grasp the posterior loop as well because this action would prevent the iris from passing between the two superior loops during insertion (Fig. 3-4). An alternative to the Clayman forceps is the model designed by Hirschman, which grasps the short vertical posts of the posterior loops of the implant where they emerge from the back surface of the optic. The right verticals of both the inferior and superior posterior loops are held with forceps for optimum stability. Thereafter, the technique of insertion is identical to the Clayman technique.

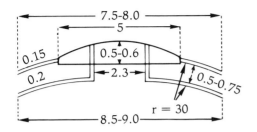

Fig. 3-2. Schematic of Binkhorst iris clip lens. All measurements are in millimeters. (From Jaffe, N.S.: Cataract surgery and its complications, ed. 3, St. Louis, 1981, The C.V. Mosby Co.)

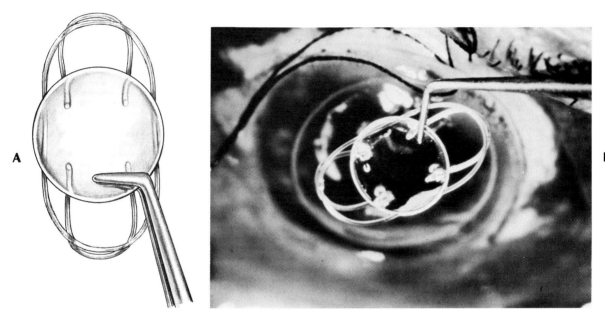

Fig. 3-3. A and **B,** Binkhorst implant held in Clayman forceps. (From Clayman, H.M.: Trans. Am. Acad. Ophthalmol. Otolaryngol. **83:**147, 1977.)

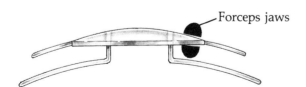

Fig. 3-4. Position of forcep jaws on optic.

Iris stromal suture. An iris stromal suture is placed at the twelve o'clock position in the iris, two thirds of the iris width distal to the pupillary margin. The bite needs to be no more than 1.0 mm and does not have to be full thickness (Fig. 3-5). The exact position of this bite changes with the variation in loop configuration from manufacturer to manufacturer. If the suture is placed too inferiorly in the iris (i.e., too close to the pupil), when it is subsequently tied the pupil will peak superiorly because it is drawn up to meet the superior loop by the tension of the suture. This is not a sight-threatening complication but is cosmetically distasteful, especially in a light-colored iris. Potentially more dangerous is the situation in which the suture is placed too high in the iris (i.e., too peripherally). In this case the implant is drawn upward and fixated in an excessively superior position, which is an invitation for chronic dislocation of the inferior loops. Also, it is worrisome to see the apex of the superior loop too close to the corneal endothelium. The effect of patient position on anterior chamber depth has been studied, and one could have justifiable concern that there would be loop-endothelial contact in the patient lying in a prone position. The problem of an intraocular lens fixated too superiorly is compounded when the spacing between the anterior and posterior loops is excessive, since the fixation suture will pull the superior

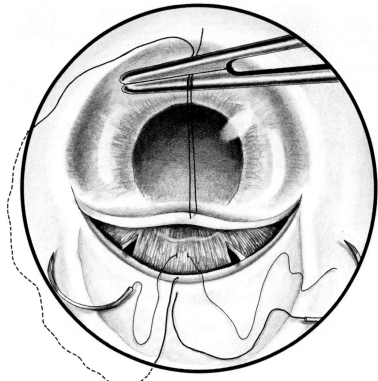

Fig. 3-5. Position of iris suture for Binkhorst iris clip lens.

loop posteriorly, which in turn will pivot the inferior loop anteriorly at the risk of the inferior corneal endothelium.

When placing the iris stromal suture, the surgeon should grasp the needle close to its heel with a fine, nonlocking needle holder, so that the bulk of the needle length is passed through the iris with the first movement of the needle holder. This makes regrasping the needle to complete the passage through the iris much easier. A nonlocking needle holder is advised, since a locking model will often recoil as the lock is released and sometimes will not release.

The point in the operation when the iris stromal suture is placed depends on whether an ICCE, ECCE, or KPE was performed. In case of an ICCE it is better to place the iris suture prior to cataract extraction because, if it was placed after extraction, the anterior hyaloid face could be ruptured by the needle's passage. When a KPE is performed, the suture is obviously placed after the cataract has been extracted and the incision sufficiently enlarged to permit IOL insertion. An ECCE is a transitional situation. The suture can be placed before or after nuclear expulsion. It can also be placed before or after I/A. Our preference is to place it after I/A (i.e., after cataract extraction) to avoid a cluttered field.

Threading the iris suture through the IOL. The cataract has been removed and the suture must be threaded through the IOL loop. The implant is held with forceps in the right hand, and the needle of the iris stromal suture is grasped with tying forceps held in the left hand. The microscope should be focused up, so that the IOL, being held at a level about the eye, is in clear view. The needle is then passed point first through the aperture of the anterior superior loop from back to front, where it is grasped by an assistant and the suture pulled through. Often an assistant is not necessary because the needle will adhere to the moistened loop. The surgeon may release the needle below the loop and regrasp it above the loop, pulling the suture through (Fig. 3-6). The next stage is IOL insertion, but prior to this the surgeon should arrange the iris suture so that it will not be snagged by the IOL during insertion and dragged into the eye (p. 219).

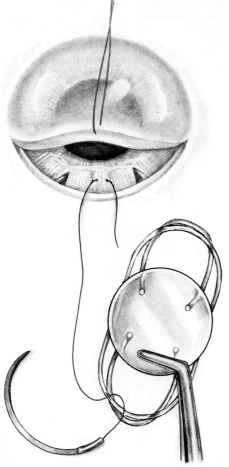

Fig. 3-6. Threading iris fixation suture through anterior superior loop of Binkhorst IOL.

IOL insertion. This will depend on the type of cataract extraction. If an ICCE was performed, sutures such as 8-0 Vicryl should be placed in the corneoscleral section at the 10 and 2 o'clock positions to effect a closed chamber. The spacing between the sutures should be 7.0 mm superior, to permit enough space for IOL insertion. The previously placed iris stromal suture is arranged on the superior sclera so that it is not obstructed by the closed chamber sutures. In an ICCE, it is at this point that the iris suture is threaded through the IOL as already described.

In case of an ECCE, the 12 o'clock suture is removed, leaving a 7.0-mm space between the remaining sutures (p. 30). As previously stated, it is our preference to place and thread the iris suture through the IOL at this point in the ECCE operation. A KPE presents a special situation, in that the incision should be enlarged from 3.0 mm to 7.0 mm by introducing corneoscleral section scissors through the original incision and enlarging it to the required size in the surgical limbus; whereupon the iris suture is placed and threaded, as noted before.

It is worth digressing at this point to discuss just how large an incision is required for implant insertion. In the case of single-plane IOLs such as the Choyce, Kelman, and Shearing-type lenses (pp. 58 and 143), a useful rule is the optic plus 1.0 mm. The optic diameter of a Binkhorst iris clip lens is 5.0 mm, but we maintain that 6.0 mm (5.0 mm + 1.0 mm) is too small for the *safe* insertion of this two-plane IOL, since the posterior loops are offset from the back surface of the IOL by 0.5 mm, giving additional bulk that must pass through the incision without stripping Descemet's membrane or snagging the iris suture. We therefore recommend a minimum incision of 7.0 mm for the Binkhorst iris clip IOL.

Returning to the method of insertion, let us assume that there is no positive vitreous pressure and that the anterior chamber holds a bubble of air with ease. The air bubble is injected into the anterior chamber through a fine cannula in sufficient quantities to fill the anterior chamber until the iris is horizontal. (A concave iris will result from too much air and will make the clipping of the inferior loops on the iris unnecessarily difficult.)

The implant is then gently slid across the anterior chamber until the inferior loops engage the inferior pupillary border, whereupon the IOL is angulated so that the posterior inferior loop slides under the iris and the superior loop over it (Fig. 3-7). The movement of the IOL is continued inferiorly until the apexes of the superior loops clear the superior pupillary border.

At this point, the direction of motion of the IOL is reversed and moved superiorly with the posterior superior loop sliding under the iris and the anterior loop over it (Fig. 3-8). The implant forceps are released and removed from the anterior chamber. This insertion is performed under an air bubble, and if any of the air was lost, a replacement aliquot should be instilled prior to the next step: tying the iris suture.

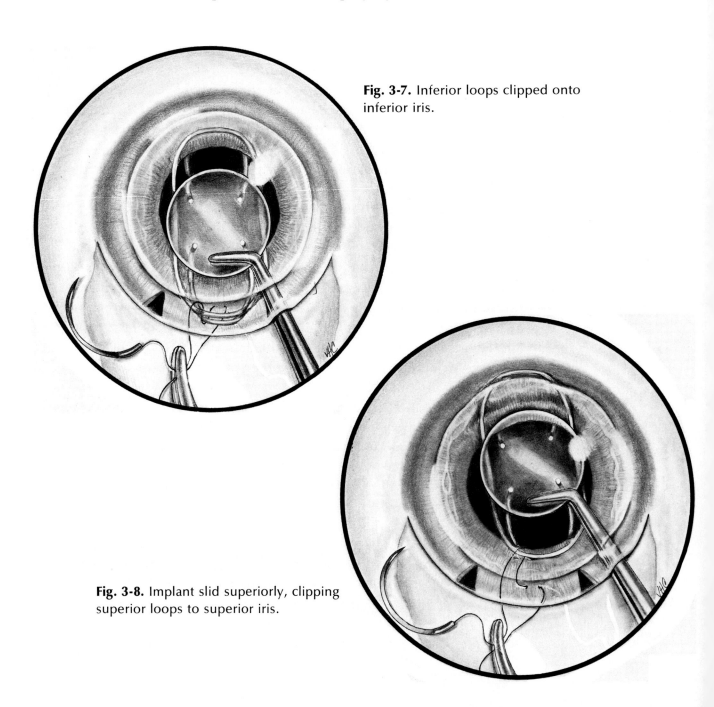

Fig. 3-7. Inferior loops clipped onto inferior iris.

Fig. 3-8. Implant slid superiorly, clipping superior loops to superior iris.

Tying of the iris suture. Acetylcholine should be injected into the anterior chamber to constrict the pupil, and any laxity in the iris suture is removed. (Fig. 3-9). The left arm of the suture is grasped with tying forceps held in the surgeon's left hand, and three overhand ties are made around another pair of tying forceps held in the right hand. The right-hand forceps then secure the right arm of the iris suture, and an assistant cuts the excess suture above the jaws of the right-hand forceps. The knot is then tightened on the superior loop of the implant. The ends of the suture should not be pulled up to the 12 o'clock position to form the knot, since this may move the IOL superiorly, dislocating the inferior loops. The surgeon's hands should tighten the knot with horizontal motions. After the first knot is tied, it is squared with two separate overhand ties. Under the air bubble the ends of the suture are trimmed close to the superior loop, and the IOL position is adjusted with a smooth spatula (Fig. 3-10). Fig. 3-11 shows, in sagittal view, an insertion and fixation of the Binkhorst iris clip lens under an air bubble.

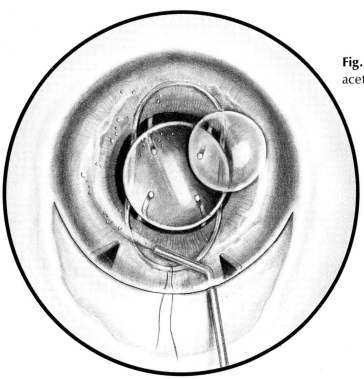

Fig. 3-9. Injection of intracameral acetylcholine.

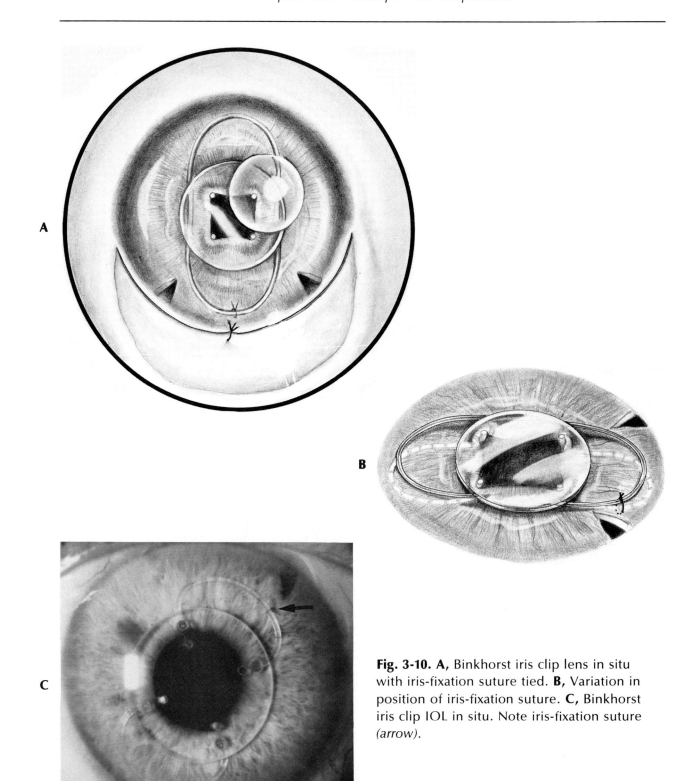

Fig. 3-10. A, Binkhorst iris clip lens in situ with iris-fixation suture tied. **B,** Variation in position of iris-fixation suture. **C,** Binkhorst iris clip IOL in situ. Note iris-fixation suture *(arrow).*

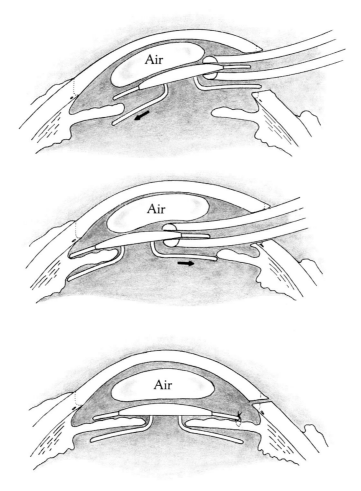

Fig. 3-11. Sagittal view of fixation and insertion of Binkhorst iris clip IOL.

Other technique

There are variations to this technique, the principal being the open-sky maneuver. Usually the implant is held in Binkhorst spring cross-action forceps, which grasp the optic (Fig. 3-12) by their own tension and are squeezed to release the implant. Realistically, these forceps are too cumbersome to use after a KPE because their configuration adds width and bulk to the optic, requiring an incision greater than 7.0 mm. This is also probably true for closed-chamber ECCE techniques.

After the cataract is extracted, the IOL, held in the forceps, is introduced into the anterior chamber and clipped onto the inferior iris (Fig. 3-13), while the cornea is retracted. The forceps are released and withdrawn from the eye (Fig. 3-14). The upper loops are positioned by using a spatula, passed horizontally between the upper loops, to depress the IOL inferiorly; meanwhile, forceps held in the left hand retract the iris superiorly so that the superior pair of loops clips onto the superior iris (Fig. 3-15). Acetylcholine is

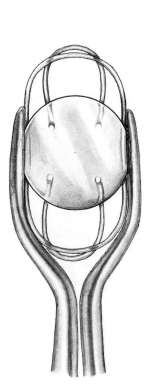

Fig. 3-12. Binkhorst iris clip IOL held in Binkhorst cross-action forceps.

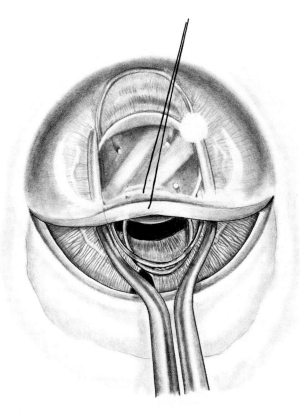

Fig. 3-13. IOL clipped onto inferior iris with Binkhorst cross-action forceps.

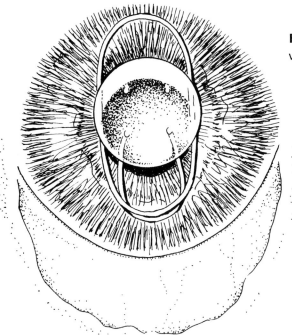

Fig. 3-14. Position of IOL after forceps withdrawn from eye.

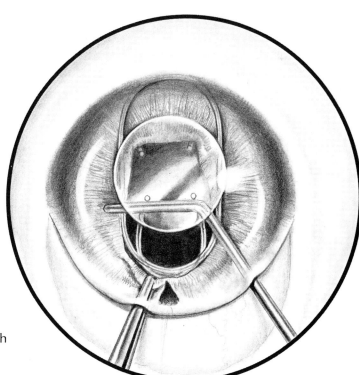

Fig. 3-15. Positioning superior loops with smooth spatula.

instilled to produce miosis. A transiridectomy suture (Fig. 3-16) is passed by a 10-0 polypropylene suture on a long taper needle.* The needle is passed from posterior to anterior, through the aperture of the peripheral iridectomy, and then through the posterior and anterior loops. The needle is cut off, the long end of the suture is tied to the short end, and the suture is cut close to the knot (Fig. 3-17). The net effect is to suspend the implant from the peripheral iridectomy (Fig. 3-18). For this technique the peripheral iridectomy should be large and situated at the 12 o'clock position.

The vogue of the open-sky technique antedated the surge in our knowledge of surgically induced trauma to the corneal endothelium. With this method there is more corneal bending and torsion of the IOL as the transiridectomy suture is passed. When there is vitreous bulge, it is an extremely difficult technique to execute, even with sodium hyaluronate. The open-sky technique is being supplanted by closed-chamber surgery.

*Ethicon no. 1789.

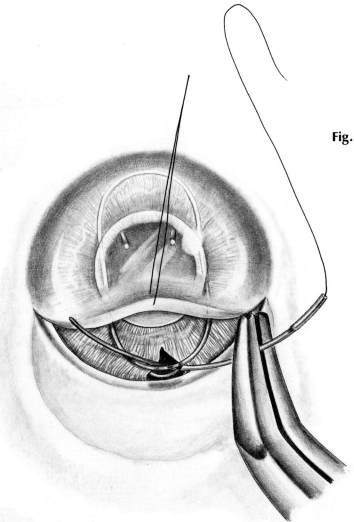

Fig. 3-16. Passage of transiridectomy suture.

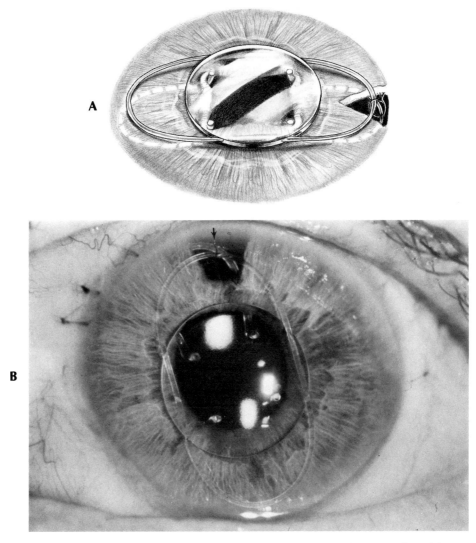

Fig. 3-17. **A,** Lens in situ with transiridectomy suture. **B,** Photographs of lens in situ. (**B** from Jaffe, N.S.: Cataract surgery and its complications, ed. 3, St. Louis, 1981, The C.V. Mosby Co.)

Fig. 3-18. Concept of transiridectomy suture.

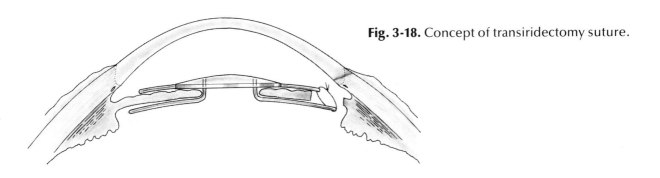

WORST MEDALLION

This implant may be used in conjunction with an ICCE or an ECCE. It is ill suited for insertion following a KPE and awkward for secondary insertion. Nevertheless, this lens, classically designed by Worst, has stood the test of time.

Description

The dimensions of the IOL vary from manufacturer to manufacturer. The model manufactured by Medical Workshop of Holland has a 5.0-mm optic surrounded eccentrically by a haptic rim with a 6.2-mm horizontal diameter. Two loops emanate from the back surface, attaining a maximum diameter of 7.6 mm (Fig. 3-19). There are two holes 2.5 mm apart in the superior optic iris through which the intracameral iris suture passes. The space between the back surface of the optic and the anterior surface of the loops is ideally 0.5 mm wide. The thickness of the optic is generally 0.5 to 0.6 mm, depending on the IOL power (Fig. 3-20).

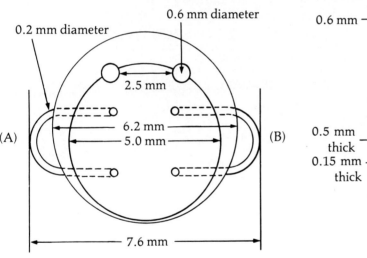

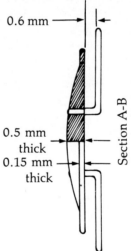

Fig. 3-19. Schematic of Worst Medallion IOL. (From Jaffe, N.S., and others: Pseudophakos, St. Louis, 1978, The C.V. Mosby Co.)

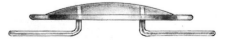

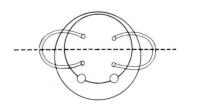

Fig. 3-20. Side view of Worst Medallion IOL.

Operation

Before cataract extraction in an ICCE and either before or after nucleus removal in an ECCE, a 9-0 polypropylene suture is placed at the 12 o'clock position through full-thickness iris (Fig. 3-21). The bite should be 2.5 mm in width (to correspond to the holes in the haptic rim) and just distal to the iris sphincter. When the pupil is dilated, the iris "accordions" on itself, and since the sphincter may not be readily identifiable, the surgeon must estimate its position. Passage of the iris suture will be made easier by straightening the needle to a ski shape. In fact, a ski-shaped needle is commercially available.* After the suture is passed, the long end is moistened so that it will adhere to the drape, and the short end (with the needle) is placed in the canthus to the surgeon's left.

*Ethicon no. 1787G.

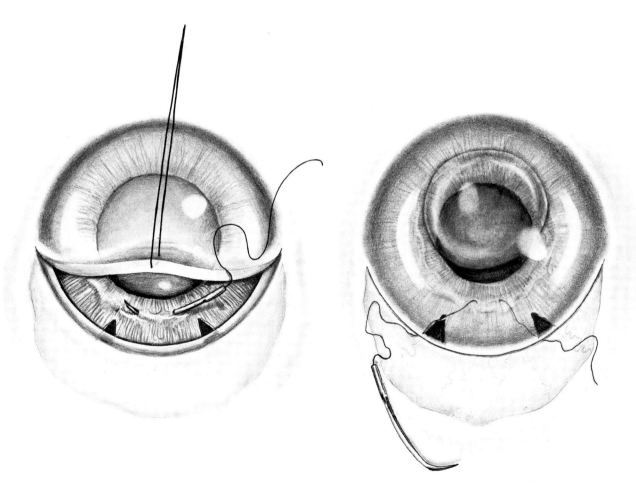

A

B

Fig. 3-21. A, Placement of iris stromal suture. **B,** Note ski-shaped needle.

The ski shape on the needle also facilitates passage of the suture through the holes of the implant. Before passing the suture, the surgeon holds the implant horizontally by the haptic rim (Fig. 3-22). The suture is secured by the forceps held in the surgeon's left hand and passed from back to front through the left hole of the implant. We recommend passing the needle heel first through the left hole (Fig. 3-23). The reason for this is that the suture and the needle are in the hole at the same time. When the needle is released from the forceps, it will not drop inferiorly by gravity but will be held within the

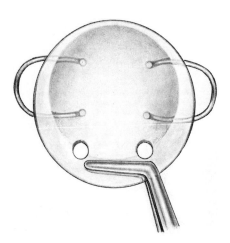

Fig. 3-22. Worst Medallion IOL held by haptic rim.

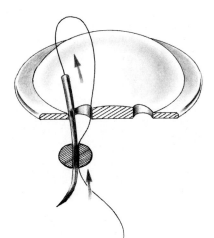

Fig. 3-23. Initial maneuver in threading iris-fixation suture through IOL.

hole by the springlike resiliency of the iris suture, so that it can be *regrasped* at the superior aspect of the hole; whereupon it is passed *point first* from front to back through the hole at the surgeon's right because in this direction gravity is helpful (Fig. 3-24). It is unusual for the needle to drop completely through the hole, since surface forces impede it. Usually about two thirds of the needle passes through. The needle is again regrasped at the inferior aspect of the IOL, the suture is drawn through, and the needle is laid at the canthus to the surgeon's right (Fig. 3-25).

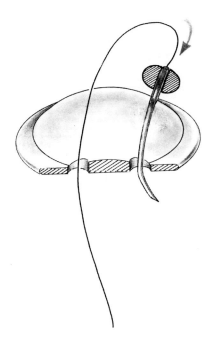

Fig. 3-24. Second maneuver in threading iris-fixation suture.

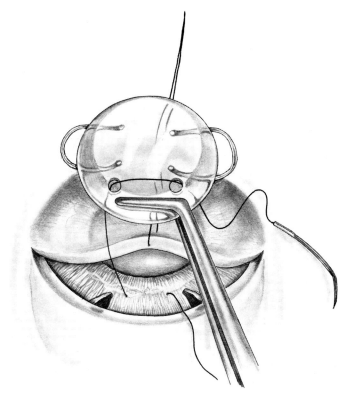

Fig. 3-25. Suture completely threaded through IOL.

It is important to arrange the suture carefully before inserting the IOL, lest the suture snag around the loops. Inserting the Medallion IOL with the loops horizontal requires at least a 9.0-mm incision. An ICCE or ECCE incision may be closed to this size or a suture may be passed through the section at the 12 o'clock position only for retraction and on the premise that the anterior chamber will not collapse. The implant is introduced with Clayman forceps into the anterior chamber under an air bubble, and the right loop is slid

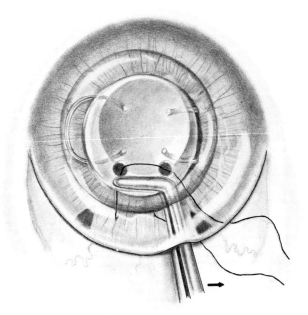

Fig. 3-26. Worst Medallion IOL with right loop inserted under iris. Arrow shows motion.

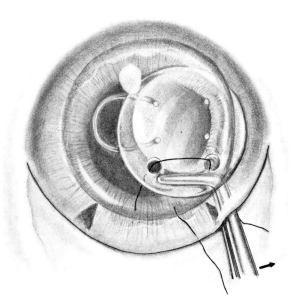

Fig. 3-27. IOL moved to right until apex of right loop clears pupillary border. Arrow shows motion.

under the iris to the right with a horizontal motion (Fig. 3-26), until the apex of the left loop clears the pupillary sphincter at the 3 o'clock position (Fig. 3-27). The implant is then slid back to the left so that the left loop slides under the iris (Fig. 3-28). The implant is centered and the forceps are removed from the eye. An ideal pupil size for insertion of the IOL is 5.0 mm. After the IOL is in situ, acetylcholine is instilled into the anterior chamber to effect miosis (Fig. 3-29).

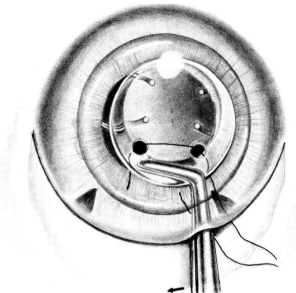

Fig. 3-28. IOL moved to left, placing left loop behind iris. Arrow shows motion.

Fig. 3-29. Lens in situ with constricted pupil.

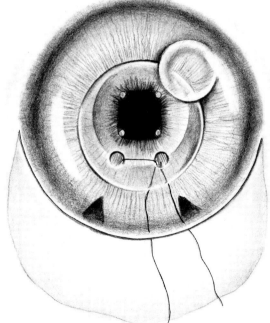

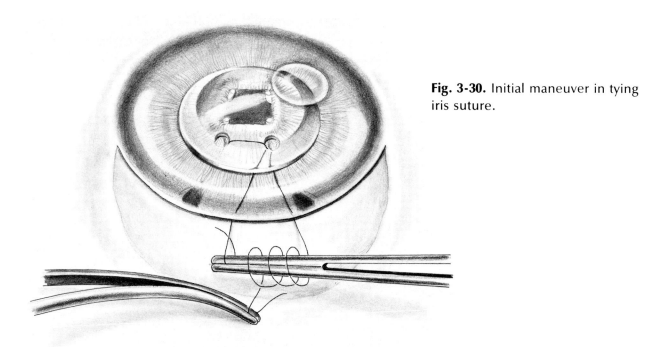

Fig. 3-30. Initial maneuver in tying iris suture.

Fig. 3-31. Squaring the knot.

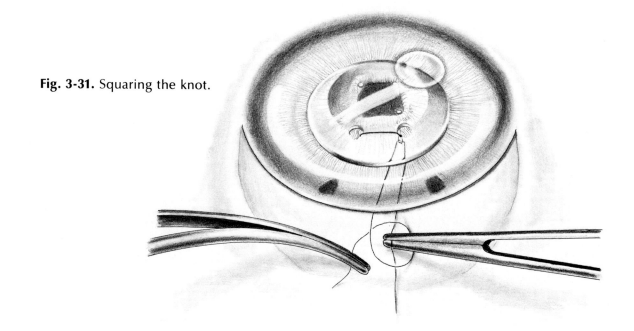

The next step is to tie the iris suture. We find it best to remove the suture's slack by pulling on the long end of the iris suture. This seems to cause less intracameral movement of the IOL than when the short end is tightened. The needle is cut from the short end of the suture and the long end tied to the short end with three overhand ties (Fig. 3-30), squared with two separate overhand ties (Fig. 3-31). The surgeon should remember to tighten the knot with equal *horizontal* forces to prevent dislocation or superior movement of the IOL with resultant haptic contact with the endothelium. The iris-fixation suture should not be excessively tight. A slight laxity of the suture is desirable and will prevent suture chafing at the edges of the haptic holes. The reader will realize at this point that, by threading the iris suture through the IOL as advocated before, the resultant knot falls between the back surface of the IOL and the front surface of the iris. This effectively traps the knot and prevents the ends of the cut suture from excoriating the endothelium. For this reason, the knot of the iris suture can be trimmed at the haptic rim rather than directly on the knot (Fig. 3-32). Closure of the incision follows, a peripheral iridectomy or iridotomy having previously been performed according to the surgeon's preference. Fig. 3-33 shows the Worst Medallion in situ.

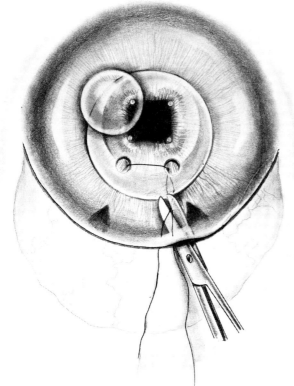

Fig. 3-32. Trimming the suture at the haptic rim.

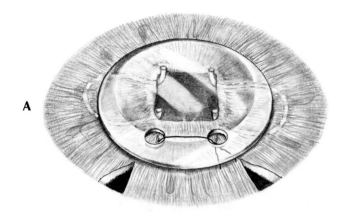

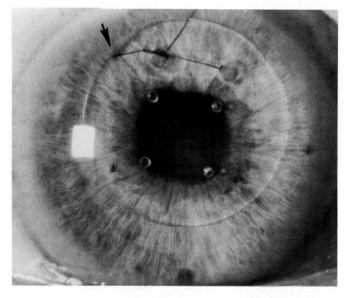

Fig. 3-33. A, Concept of Worst Medallion IOL in situ. **B,** Photograph of Worst Medallion in situ. Note iris suture *(arrow).* (**B** from Jaffe, N.S., and others: Pseudophakos, St. Louis, 1978, The C.V. Mosby Co.)

Comments

Realistically, the Worst Medallion is a very difficult lens to insert in the face of a substantial iris bulge. Some surgeons advocate inserting the lens through a 7.0- to 8.0-mm incision with the loops vertical and then rotating the IOL to the horizontal position. This is the sort of intracameral gymnastics that, although feasible, is hazardous to the corneal endothelium and runs the risk of snagging the suture (p. 219). Furthermore, the initial step of the closed-chamber technique is often open-sky because the horizontal IOL loop diameter and the implant bulk may preclude sliding the IOL into the anterior chamber without corneal retraction. A pure open-sky technique is preferred by some loupe surgeons who operate with an oblique (as opposed to vertical) view of the anterior chamber through the operating microscope (Fig. 3-34).

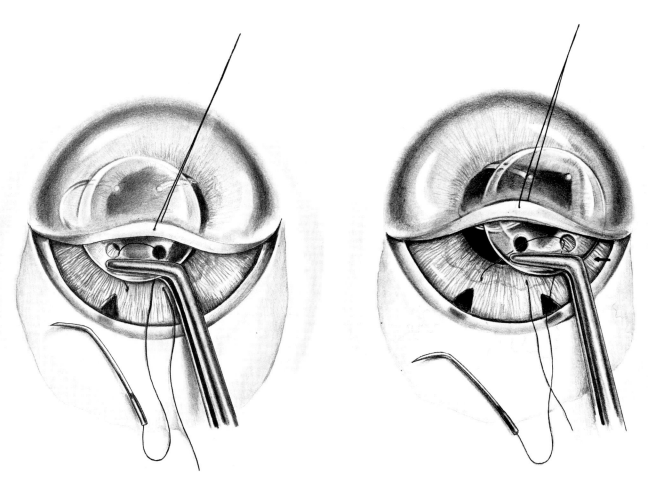

B

Fig. 3-34. A, Open-sky placement of right loop under iris. **B,** Open-sky placement of left loop under iris. Arrow shows motion of forceps.

FYODOROV-BINKHORST LENS
Description

The Fyodorov-Binkhorst lens consists of a 5.0-mm optic with two sets of haptic loops. The axes of the loops are at right angles to each other. One set of loops is offset from the back surface of the optic and is placed posteriorly to the iris, and the other set is anterior (Fig. 3-35). The lens may be inserted with the posterior loops either horizontally or vertically placed behind the iris.

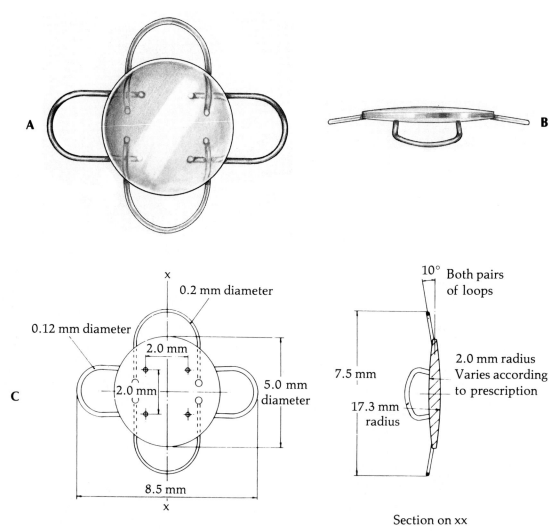

Fig. 3-35. A, Fyodorov-Binkhorst IOL. **B,** Fyodorov-Binkhorst IOL (side view). **C,** Schematic of Fyodorov-Binkhorst IOL. (**C** from Jaffe, N.S., and others: Pseudophakos, St. Louis, 1978, The C.V. Mosby Co.)

Operation

To insert the loops vertically posterior to the iris, the optic is grasped with Clayman forceps close to the origin of the superior posterior loop (Fig. 3-36). Because the horizontal haptic diameter is approximately 8.6 mm, this lens is ill suited for insertion after a KPE; the incision would be excessively large. Furthermore, in an ICCE and an ECCE a closed-chamber technique is difficult because an 8.0- to 9.0-mm incision is required for the insertion of this two-plane, horizontal haptic lens. A soft eye is mandatory for this technique.

The cornea is carefully retracted, and the implant is slid into the anterior chamber. The inferior posterior loop is slid under the inferior iris, and the implant is moved inferiorly, until the apex of the superior posterior loop clears the superior pupillary margin (Fig. 3-37). The implant is then slid su-

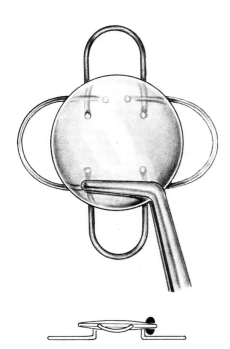

Fig. 3-36. Fyodorov-Binkhorst IOL held in forceps.

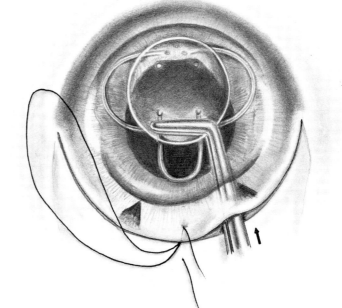

Fig. 3-37. IOL's inferior loop slid under inferior iris. Arrow shows motion.

periorly so that the superior posterior loop comes into position behind the iris (Fig. 3-38). The forceps are then released and withdrawn from the eye. Acetylcholine is instilled into the anterior chamber to induce miosis (Fig. 3-39). The lens is now in situ (Fig. 3-40).

To insert this lens with the horizontal loops posterior to the iris, the optic should be held at the origin of the superior anterior loop. The cornea must be retracted to allow the lens into the anterior chamber, whereupon it is slid to the right so that the right horizontal loop passes under the iris (Fig. 3-41). This motion is continued to the right until the apex of the left horizontal loop clears the left pupillary margin. The implant is then slid left (Fig. 3-42), placing the left horizontal loop behind the iris. Miosis is obtained as already cited (Fig. 3-43), and peripheral iridectomies are performed according to the surgeon's preference.

Comments

We have several general comments on the Fyodorov-Binkhorst lens. First, it is easy to insert into a soft eye with a vacuous anterior chamber and a 5.0- to 6.0-mm pupil. It is a lens very difficult to insert with positive vitreous pressure. Second, the lens is easier to insert with the *vertical* loops posterior to the iris into a soft eye with a pupil that has constricted after cataract extraction. The reason is that iris retraction will be required to place the posterior loops, and it is easier to retract the iris at the 12 o'clock position than at the 3 o'clock position (which would be necessary if the horizontal loops were posterior to the iris). Third, the Fyodorov-Binkhorst lens has a predilection for rotatory pseudophacodonesis and dislocation. For this reason some surgeons use an iris-fixation suture that is placed in the iris stroma as described for the Binkhorst iris clip lens (p. 86). Naturally, in this case the suture would have to be threaded through the *anterior* superior loop, which means that the horizontal loops, of necessity, would be posterior to the iris.

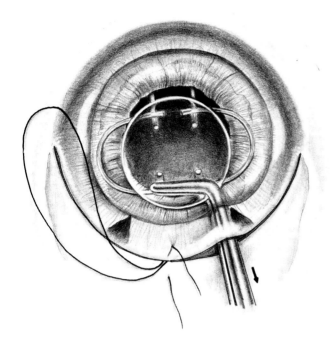

Fig. 3-38. IOL's superior loop is positioned behind superior iris. Arrow shows motion.

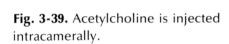

Fig. 3-39. Acetylcholine is injected intracamerally.

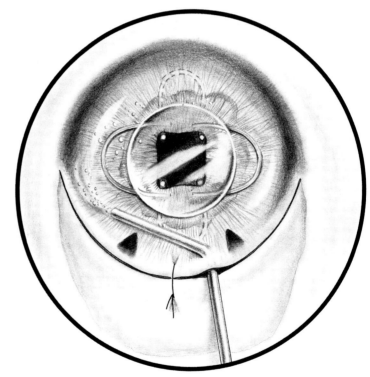

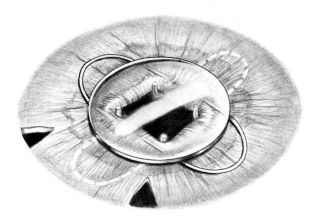

Fig. 3-40. Fyodorov-Binkhorst IOL in situ with vertical loops posterior to iris.

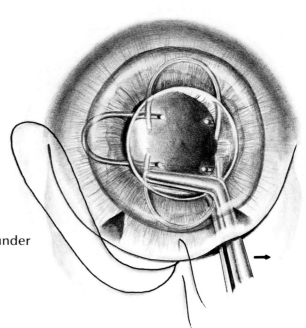

Fig. 3-41. Right horizontal loop slid under iris. Arrow shows motion.

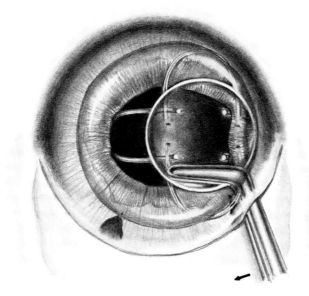

Fig. 3-42. Left horizontal loop being positioned. Arrow shows motion.

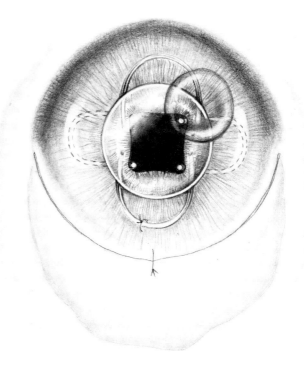

Fig. 3-43. Fyodorov-Binkhorst IOL in situ with horizontal loops posterior to iris (iridectomies not shown). Iris-fixation suture secures anterior superior loop.

COPELAND LENS

The Copeland lens is unique among iris-fixated lenses for three reasons. First, the optic is iris plane, in contradistinction to the other iris-fixated lenses already described, in which the optic is prepupillary. Second, the Copeland lens is of one-piece design, being fixated with haptic feet rather than with loops of a material dissimilar to the optic. Third, the Copeland lens is *single plane*, i.e., without haptic loops offset from the back surface. It can be inserted through a smaller incision than can the other iris-fixated lenses because of its single-plane design. Furthermore, the single-plane construction permits the lens to slide into the anterior chamber with minimal corneal retraction, but an 8.0-mm incision at least is required for insertion—so the advantage of a KPE is partially lost.

Description

The Copeland lens is cruciate with a 4.0-mm planoconvex optic in the center. The overall foot diameter is 9.0 mm and the width of the feet is 2.5 mm. The optic thickness varies with the lens power; a 17.62-D lens is 0.4 mm thick (Fig. 3-44). Variations in foot diameter and width can be obtained on special order from the manufacturer.

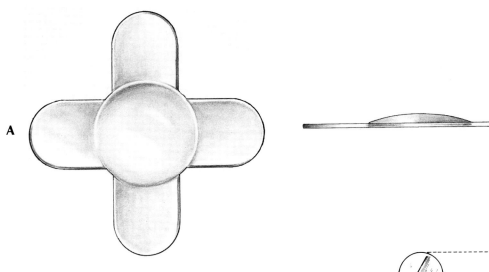

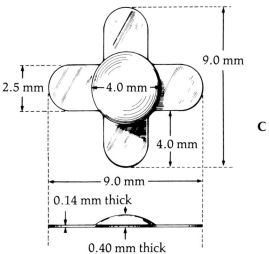

Fig. 3-44. A, Copeland IOL. **B,** Copeland IOL (side view). **C,** Schematic of Copeland IOL. (**C** from Jaffe, N.S., and others: Pseudophakos, St. Louis, 1978, The C.V. Mosby Co.)

Operation

As with the other iris-fixation lenses, a 5.0-mm pupil is ideal. The lens may be inserted with the vertical feet posterior to the iris and the horizontal feet anterior (Fig. 3-45, *A*), or vice versa (Fig. 3-45, *B*). In the former case, the lens is grasped by the right horizontal foot and slid into the anterior chamber under an air bubble. The inferior foot is slid under the inferior iris (Fig. 3-46) and held in that position while the superior iris is retracted over the superior foot (Fig. 3-47). The lens is then in situ (Fig. 3-48), and acetylcholine is instilled in the anterior chamber for miosis (Fig. 3-49). Insertion is easier when the feet are placed slightly obliquely behind the iris, as shown in the illustrations.

To place the horizontal feet behind the iris, the implant is held by the superior foot, and introduced into the anterior chamber. The right foot is slid under the iris at the 9 o'clock position. The iris is retracted at the 2 o'clock position adjacent to the left foot, and the implant is released. Miosis is obtained.

A "Frisbee" maneuver, to engage the superior foot when the verticals are posterior to the iris or the left foot when the horizontals are posterior, is often difficult because of the overall 9.0-mm foot diameter and the inflexibility of the feet. For this reason we advocate iris retraction.

Comments

The Copeland lens is relatively easy to insert and requires no fixation suture. It single-plane design permits its insertion with minimal corneal retraction, thus preserving the air bubble. The lens is also extremely resistant to dislocation. For these reasons the lens is especially well suited for the novice implant surgeon.

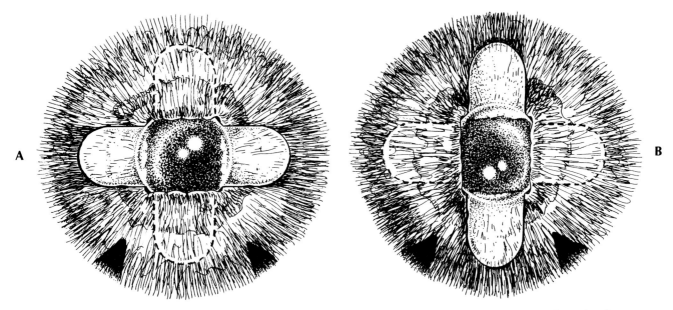

Fig. 3-45. A, Copeland in situ with vertical feet posterior to iris. B, Copeland in situ with horizontal feet posterior to iris.

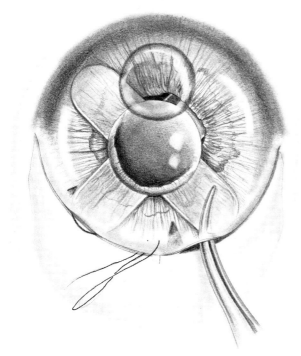

Fig. 3-46. Inferior foot slid under iris slightly obliquely.

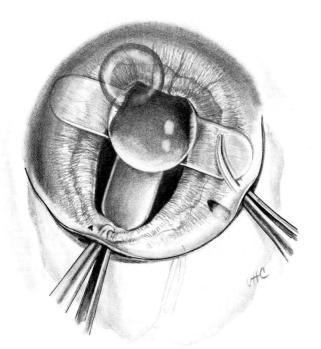

Fig. 3-47. Iris retracted over superior foot.

Fig. 3-48. Copeland lens in situ with vertical loops posterior to iris.

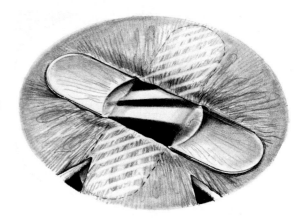

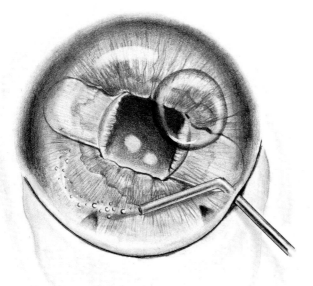

Fig. 3-49. Instillation of acetylcholine for miosis.

FYODOROV SPUTNIK LENS

This lens evolved from the Fyodorov-Binkhorst lens, substituting anterior pintles for anterior loops.

Description

The Fyodorov Sputnik lens implant consists of a 5.0-mm optic with three loops emanating from the optic's back surface and offset approximately 0.5 mm from the posterior plane of the optic. The distance between the apexes of adjacent loops is 8.0 mm (Fig. 3-50). The anterior struts (or pintles) arise at the lateral edge of the implant and are positioned anterior to the iris to give the lens stability (Fig. 3-51).

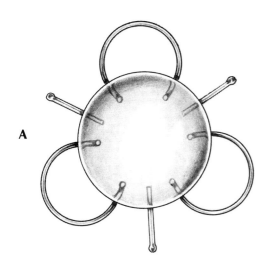

A

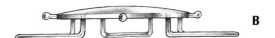

B

Fig. 3-50. A, Fyodorov Sputnik IOL. **B,** Fyodorov Sputnik IOL (side view).

Fig. 3-51. Fyodorov Sputnik in situ. (From Jaffe, N.S., and others: Pseudophakos, St. Louis, 1978, The C.V. Mosby Co.)

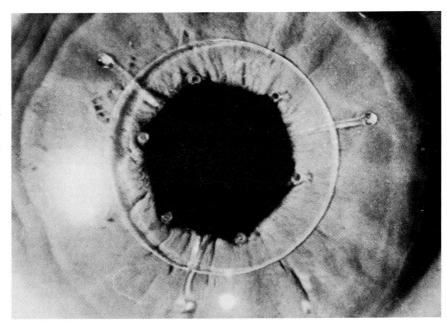

Operation

This lens may be inserted after either an ICCE or ECCE, but the total diameter and two-plane construction of the lens negates the advantages of small-incision surgery.

With a concave iris diaphragm the Sputnik lens, held in a Binkhorst lens forceps, which grasps the edge of the implant, may be inserted by open-sky technique. A pupil with a diameter of at least 6.0 mm is essential for this technique. The cornea is retracted, and the inferior loop of the implant is slid un-

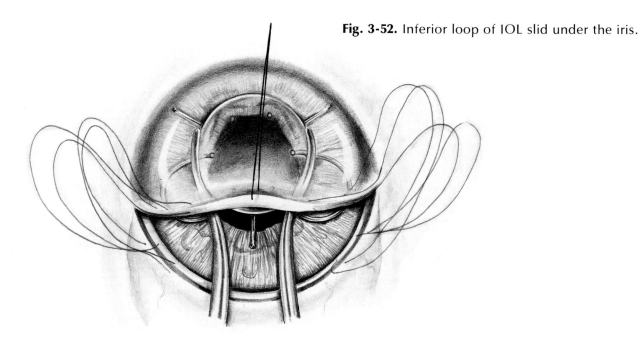

Fig. 3-52. Inferior loop of IOL slid under the iris.

der the iris at the 6 o'clock position (Fig. 3-52). Two loops remain anterior to the iris in the approximate horizontal position. The lens is then slid to the surgeon's left so that the apex of the right-hand loop clears the pupillary border and is slid under the iris into the 9 o'clock position (Fig. 3-53). The motion is continued to the surgeon's right until the apex of the left loop clears the pupillary margin, whereupon it is slid under the iris at the 3 o'clock position (Fig. 3-54); the lens is in position. Miosis is obtained with acetylcholine, and the resultant pupil is hexagonal (Fig. 3-55).

Fig. 3-53. Right loop slid under right lateral iris after loop apex clears pupillary margin. Arrow shows motion.

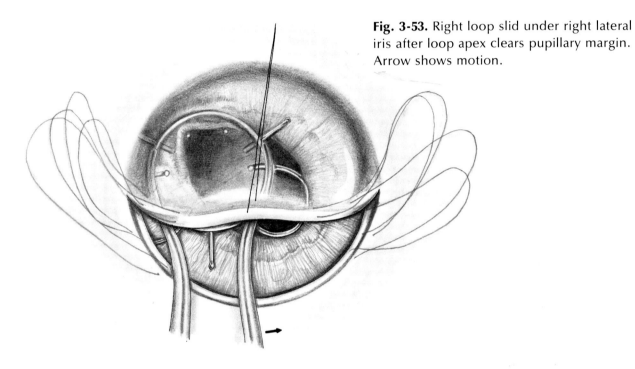

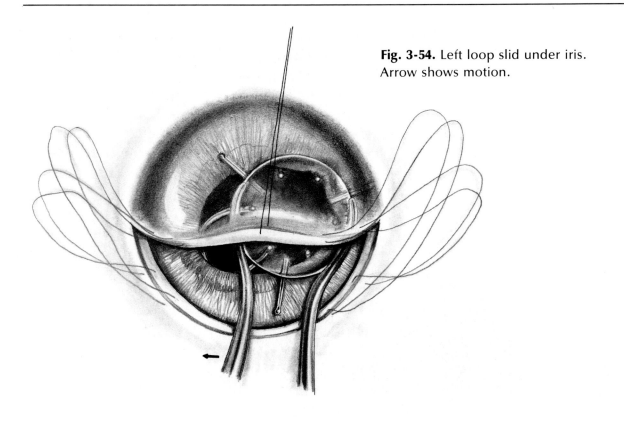

Fig. 3-54. Left loop slid under iris. Arrow shows motion.

Fig. 3-55. Fyodorov Sputnik IOL in situ, showing relation of loops to pintles. Note hexagonal pupil.

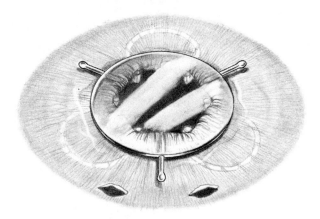

Comments

The Sputnik lens is very difficult to insert in the presence of a substantial vitreous bulge, and the procedure should either be aborted, or sodium hyaluronate (p. 272) should be used. In the event of a mild vitreous bulge, in which nonetheless a small air bubble can be retained in the anterior chamber, the lens can be inserted with a modified closed-chamber technique and *three* preplaced sutures. The lens is eased into the anterior chamber, replacing the air bubble as required, and the inferior loop is lid under the iris. A 5.0- to 6.0-mm pupil is desirable. The preplaced sutures are now tied, and balanced saline or air is introduced into the anterior chamber, which is deepened to aphakic depth. Additional sutures are added as required for a watertight closure. A flat spatula is inserted through the incision behind the optic but anterior to the right loop. The spatula actually rests against the vertical portion of the offset posterior loop. The lens is displaced to the left until the apex of the right loop clears the pupillary margin, at which point slight posterior pressure on the loop by the spatula with a right lateral motion will position the right loop posterior to the iris. The spatula is then repositioned behind the optic and anterior to the left loop. The lens is moved to the right, and as the apex of the left loop clears the pupillary border, gentle posterior pressure is applied, and the left loop "pops" behind the iris. The spatula is withdrawn, and acetylcholine is instilled for miosis.

The popularity of this lens and all iris-fixated IOLs is declining in the United States.

Four
Iridocapsular intraocular lenses

GENERAL PRINCIPLES

Over the years several implants have been designed for iridocapsular fixation. The two primary lenses are the Binkhorst iridocapsular (2-loop) and the Worst Platina clip IOLs. *Iridocapsular* implies that both the posterior capsule and the iris are involved in IOL fixation and centration.

Some modifications of the ECCE procedure have been advocated by proponents of these lenses. The most important involves the anterior capsulectomy, which has been performed in a variety of shapes, including the "Xmas tree" (Fig. 4-1), or more usually an H-shaped configuration (Fig. 4-2). After the nucleus and cortex are removed, the H capsulectomy results in inferior and superior capsular flaps, or scrolls, *behind* which the respective loops of the IOL are implanted into the capsular bag. This is to enhance fixation, a recurring theme with iridocapsular-fixated IOLs (p. 134). The theory is that the capsular epithelium will adhere to the IOL loops and/or posterior capsule, thus securing the IOL; whether it has merit is speculative. Fig. 4-3 shows a Binkhorst iridocapsular IOL, 4 days after implantation, nicely adherent to the posterior capsule without the benefit of capsular flaps. Fixation may be an interaction solely between the IOL loops and posterior capsule with residual cortex as the glue.

Removal of the nucleus, either manually with an ECCE or ultrasonically in a KPE, can be more difficult when capsular flaps are present. With an ECCE the incision should be sufficient to allow the surgeon to expose the superior pole of the nucleus with capsular retraction, should it be necessary. As we have previously discussed (pp. 26, 28), if the egress of the nucleus from the anterior chamber is restrained by an inadequate incision, miotic pupil, or inadequate capsulectomy, the consequences can be disastrous. An H capsulectomy can make nuclear prolapse in a KPE exceedingly difficult. If a posterior-chamber KPE is planned, the flaps may impede "sculpting" of the nucleus (p. 48) and may be inadvertently shredded when the machine is turned to position 3 (ultrasound).

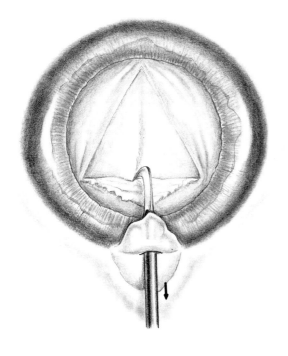

Fig. 4-1. "Xmas tree" anterior capsulectomy.

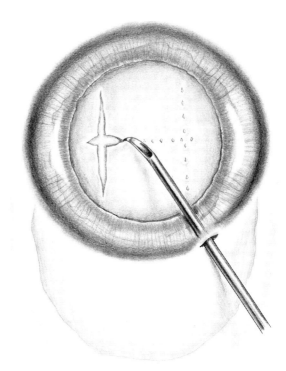

Fig. 4-2. Technique of H anterior capsulectomy.

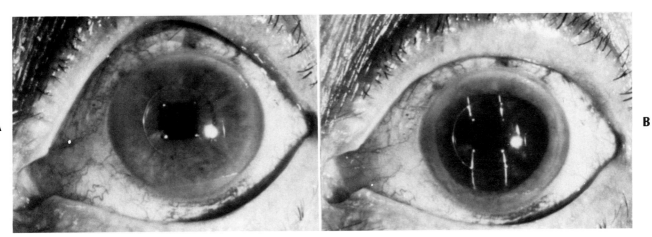

Fig. 4-3. A, Binkhorst 2-loop iridocapsular IOL, 4 days postoperatively. **B,** Same eye dilated; note capsular fixation. (From Jaffe, N.S.: Cataract surgery and its complications, ed. 3, St. Louis, 1981, The C.V. Mosby Co.)

In the ECCE or KPE with capsular flaps just described, some difficulties may be experienced in the I/A phase of the operation. The flaps tend to clog the aspiration orifice and may not release even when the surgeon switches from foot position 2 (I/A) to position 1 (irrigation only). If this occurs, the aspiration line should be "milked" toward the handpiece by an assistant, to induce a counterflow at the aspiration orifice, which releases the entrapped capsular flap. Entrapment of capsular flaps recurs with annoying frequency and can be largely obviated by a smooth spatula in the left hand (Fig. 1-47). This instrument is inserted at the 2 o'clock position, through the incision in the case of an ECCE or through a second incision (pp. 48 and 49) if a KPE is performed. The spatula is used to lift the flaps as the I/A handpiece, in position 1 (irrigation), is insinuated below them into the capsular cul-de-sac. The foot pedal is depressed to position 2 (I/A) and the cortex is aspirated. This maneuver may have to be repeated several times, until all the cortex is evacuated. Realistically, the use of the spatula is easiest when the inferior capsular flap is being retracted. Access to the superior capsular cul-de-sac, however, is difficult when a superior capsular flap is present. Instead of a spatula, a microhook (Fig. 5-24, *A*) may be more beneficial. This is inserted adjacent to the I/A handpiece through the same incision. The capsule is hooked superiorly, exposing the contents of the superior capsular cul-de-sac, which are aspirated. In spite of best efforts, it is sometimes not feasible to achieve this; the surgeon should not risk superior zonular dialysis or capsular rupture through dogged persistence. Residual superior cortex sometimes drops into the pupillary aperture (p. 268), sometimes swells, as we will discuss with the Worst Platina, but usually does nothing except participate in Soemmering ring formation.

Advocates of nonautomated ECCE state that with their techniques the iris and capsular flap can be retracted as required, and that capsular cul-de-sac contents can be removed with a variety of aspiration tips. It is our opinion that these methods do not remove cortex as well as an automated closed-chamber system, except perhaps in the hands of an elite few. Moreover, we believe that the use of capsular flaps adds an unnecessary complexity to the operation. We agree that iridocapsular IOLs should be placed in the capsular bag (Fig. 4-4) and achieve this by making the "can opener" capsulectomy (p. 24) of smaller diameter. This serves to delineate the edges of the anterior capsule without having *mobile* flaps to impede cortical aspiration.

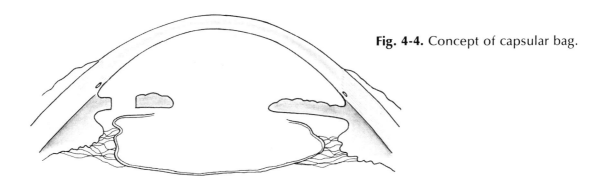

Fig. 4-4. Concept of capsular bag.

BINKHORST 2-LOOP IRIDOCAPSULAR IOL

This lens can be inserted only after an ECCE or a KPE. It evolved from the Binkhorst iris clip (4-loop) IOL (p. 83) and was first used in 1965.

Description

The lens has a 5.0-mm diameter optic and is 0.5 to 0.6-mm thick, depending on dioptric power. Most manufacturers produce a lens in a planoconvex configuration with the convex surface anterior. Some biconvex models are available. Two loops originate from the back surface of the optic in opposite directions and have a diameter from apex to apex of approximately 8.0 mm. The loops are angled posteriorly 10 to 15 degrees, generally conforming to the contour of the posterior iris in a phakic eye (Fig. 4-5). Originally the loops were metallic, either platinum-iridium or titanium; now plastics are used. Polypropylene is the loop material favored by most manufacturers, although nylon 6 (Supramid) is also used.

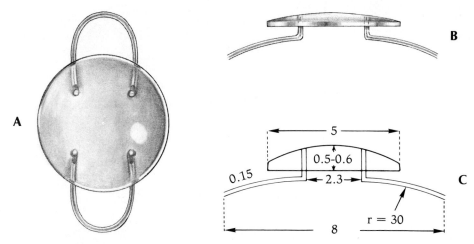

Fig. 4-5. A, Binkhorst iridocapsular IOL. **B,** Binkhorst iridocapsular IOL (side view). **C,** Schematic of Binkhorst iridocapsular IOL. (**C** from Jaffe, N.S.: Cataract surgery and its complications, ed. 3, St. Louis, 1981, The C.V. Mosby Co.)

Operation

After the cataract extraction the incision must be opened to the appropriate size. Both IOLs described in this chapter are two-plane (i.e., the loops are offset from the optic's back surface by approximately 0.5 mm), and the incision must accommodate both the maximum IOL width *and thickness.* In the case of the Binkhorst iridocapsular IOL, we suggest 7.0 mm, which represents 5.0 mm (optic diameter) + 2.0 mm. Following the techniques presented in Chapter 1, removal of the 12 o'clock suture in an ECCE (p. 30) will give the desired incision. A KPE incision may be enlarged to 7.0 mm (p. 46). To insert the IOL, grasp the right vertical posts of both the inferior and superior loops at their origin from the posterior surface of the optic, with Kelman-McPherson or Hirschman forceps, or the optic rim with Clayman forceps (Fig. 4-6). The implant should then be slid into the anterior chamber under an air bubble. Its two-plane construction pries the incision farther apart than a single-plane IOL, so the air bubble may be lost. In that case, additional aliquots of air should be instilled as required. The inferior loop is inserted into the inferior capsular bag (Fig. 4-7). If capsular flaps were used, the in-

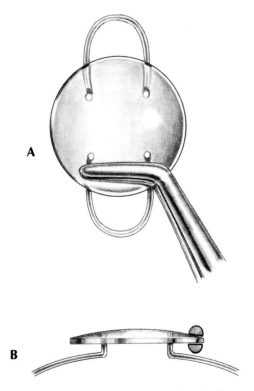

Fig. 4-6. A, Optic rim grasped with forceps. **B,** Side view of IOL held with Clayman forceps.

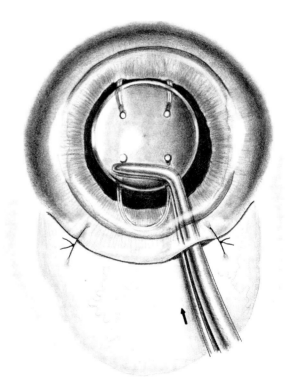

Fig. 4-7. Inferior loop of IOL slid under iris and into inferior capsular bag.

ferior flap may have to be manipulated with a spatula, as already described, to prevent it from folding in on itself or from floating *under* the advancing inferior loop, in which case the inferior loop would not be in the capsular bag. When the apex of the superior loop has cleared the pupillary margin, the IOL is slid superiorly (Fig. 4-8), positioning the superior loop in the superior capsular cul-de-sac. The implant forceps are then released and withdrawn from the eye. Alternatively, the superior loop can be positioned with either a Hirschman or a smooth spatula held in the right hand and Hoskin forceps or an iris hook held in the left hand (Fig 4-9). Intracameral acetylcholine is instilled for miosis (Fig. 4-10).

A minor point concerns the use of the right-handed spatula. Following a KPE it is advantageous to use the Hirschman spatula. This instrument has a notch at its tip and is maneuverable within the constraints of the KPE's 7.0-mm incision. With the right-handed instrument the implant is displaced inferiorly to permit the apex of the superior loop to fall back behind the superior iris and the superior anterior capsular margin (or the superior capsular flap, if present). This is best executed with a well-dilated pupil, and following IOL positioning, miosis is induced with intracameral acetylcholine. When adequate pupillary dilatation is not obtainable the hook or forceps held in the left hand are used to retract iris and anterior capsule as the IOL is displaced inferiorly with the spatula, whereupon the superior loop is positioned, and miosis is obtained. Sometimes the surgeon cannot be completely sure if the superior loop is in the superior capsular bag and should *not* subject the eye to excessive manipulation to find out. Although both loops in the capsular bag are desirable one loop will generally suffice for fixation.

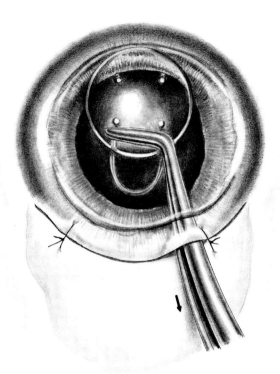

Fig. 4-8. Implant slid superiorly once apex of superior loop has cleared the pupillary margin.

Fig. 4-9. Positioning of superior loop of Binkhorst iridocapsular IOL with spatula and forceps.

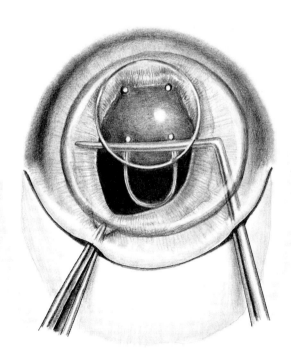

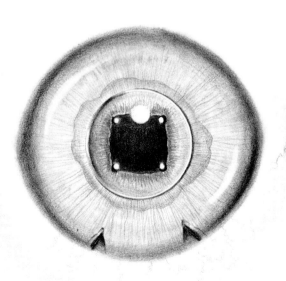

Fig. 4-10. Miotic pupil with IOL in situ.

Open-sky insertion of the Binkhorst iridocapsular IOL requires a full-size incision and therefore would completely negate the advantages of a KPE. With an ECCE the cornea is retracted and the implant grasped with Binkhorst cross-action forceps, so that the IOL can be inserted with the loops vertically or obliquely placed (Fig. 4-11). The inferior loop is slid under the corresponding iris and into the capsular bag (Figs. 4-12 and 4-13). If the pupil is large enough, the inferior motion is continued until the apex of the superior loop clears the adjacent iris, at which time the IOL is slid superiorly, so that the superior loop rests posterior to the iris and, ideally, in the superior capsular cul-de-sac. We use the word *ideally* because, when the anterior chamber is decompressed, as with iris retraction, the margins of the intracameral anatomy are indistinct and the potential spaces between them, e.g., between anterior and posterior capsules, are collapsed. Therefore loop insertion between them is difficult and probably fortuitous when it does occur.

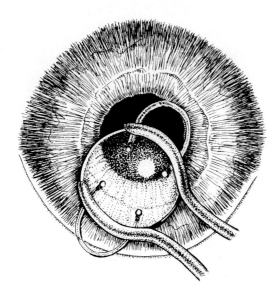

Fig. 4-11. Binkhorst iridocapsular IOL obliquely held in Binkhorst cross-action forceps.

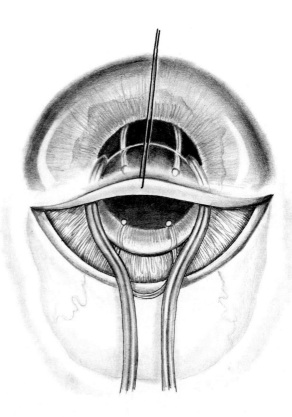

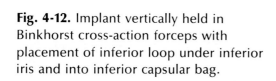

Fig. 4-12. Implant vertically held in Binkhorst cross-action forceps with placement of inferior loop under inferior iris and into inferior capsular bag.

When the pupil constricts before an IOL insertion, a bimanual technique is used. If the IOL has been held obliquely in the cross-action forceps, iris can be retracted over the superior loop (Fig. 4-14) while the IOL is steadied with the forceps. The forceps are then released. This can be difficult when the IOL is vertically held. If it is, the cross-action forceps are released after the inferior loop is in position. The implant is steadied with a spatula while the iris is lifted over the superior loop by forceps held in the left hand (Fig. 4-9). We do not feel that open-sky insertion is compatible with contemporary IOL surgery, except under extenuating circumstances. The concept of the lens in situ is shown in Fig. 4-15.

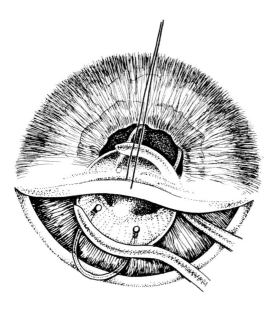

Fig. 4-13. Implant obliquely held in forceps, showing placement of inferior loop under inferior iris and into inferior capsular bag.

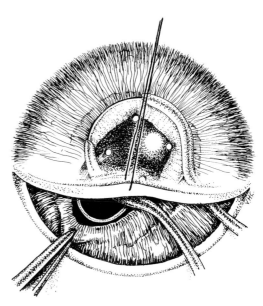

Fig. 4-14. Iris retracted over superior loop of Binkhorst iridocapsular IOL, as IOL is steadied with cross-action forceps.

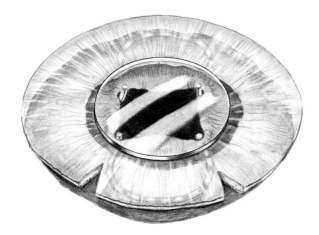

Fig. 4-15. Binkhorst iridocapsular lens in situ.

Compared to other types of IOL, the postoperative regimen is somewhat onerous with the Binkhorst iridocapsular IOL. Keeping in mind the concept of fixation, the surgeon instills topical miotics in the first 72 hours postoperatively to immobilize and center the IOL. Thereafter, mydriasis is required to break iris adhesions. The goal is capsular fixation without iris synechiae, and to this purpose mydriasis and miosis are alternatingly used in the subsequent 2 weeks. If the implant decenters inferiorly with pupillary dilatation, capsular fixation has not been achieved, and the lens is dropping by gravity. In this case, miotics should be continued for several more days before mydriasis is again attempted.

Comments

Notwithstanding capsular flaps, insertion into the capsular bag, and scrupulous postoperative care, there is failure of capsular fixation in approximately 10% of cases. Some are dislocations. These patients can be maintained with chronic topical miotic therapy, but this becomes tiresome for many patients who lapse into noncompliance, and it is not without complication (p. 264). Some surgeons have attempted to augment capsular fixation by using an iris-fixation suture to immobilize the IOL partially until capsular fixation can take place. An iris-fixation suture would also limit the potential for IOL dislocation and confine its effects to those attributable to the inferior loop. An iris-fixation suture can be placed once the lens is in situ. A 10-0 polypropylene suture (p. 86) is passed through the iris stroma, around one arm of the superior loop, and out through the adjacent stroma, where it is tied and trimmed. Alternately, the suture can be passed through the margin of the peripheral iridectomy and around an arm of the superior loop, from back to front, whereupon the suture is tied and trimmed.

The insertion of the Binkhorst iridocapsular IOL is often facilitated by the Sheets glide, which is discussed in Chapter 10.

WORST PLATINA IOL

This IOL has features designed to remedy the fixation problems oc-
curring in some patients who have a Binkhorst iridocapsular lens. The Worst
Platina has the same optic as the Worst Medallion IOL (p. 98).

Description

The optic is 5.0 mm and is incorporated onto a 6.2-mm–diameter haptic
carrier. The superior bore holes in the IOL are not used in this technique.
The lens is inserted vertically, and two plastic loops (nylon or polypropylene), oriented vertically, arise from the back surface of the implant. The loops
are *unequal* in length, the inferior loop being approximately 3.5 mm in length
and the superior loop 2.7 mm (Fig. 4-16). As with the Worst Medallion, the
loops are offset from the back of the optic by 0.6 mm, making this a two-plane
IOL (Fig. 4-17). The thickness of the optic varies with IOL power and aver-

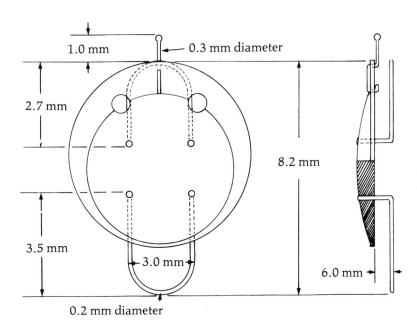

Fig. 4-16. Schematic of Worst
Platina IOL. (From Jaffe, N.S., and
others: Pseudophakos, St. Louis,
1978, The C.V. Mosby Co.)

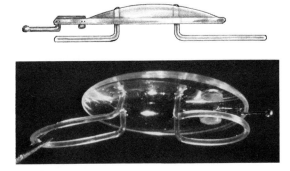

Fig. 4-17. Worst Platina lens in side view.
Note offset posterior loops, which make this
a 2-plane IOL.

ages 0.5 mm. The distinguishing feature of this IOL is a platinum wire originating from the superior edge of the IOL haptic and extending 1.0 or 2.0 mm in the same plane as the haptic (Fig. 4-18). The platinum wire concept gave the name *platina* to this IOL, although some manufacturers have substituted a plastic stave, usually polypropylene, for the platinum wire. Whether wire or plastic stave, the purpose of this appendage is to function as a clip by being bent through the aperture of the peripheral iridectomy and around the superior loop after the IOL is in situ (Fig. 4-19).

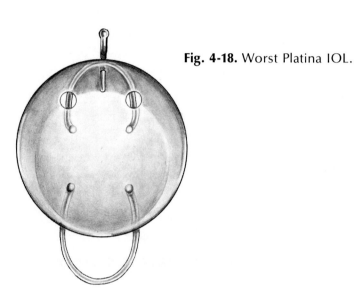

Fig. 4-18. Worst Platina IOL.

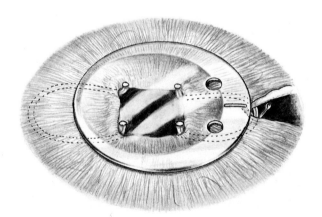

Fig. 4-19. Concept of Worst Platina with superior stave bent to form a clip around superior posterior loop.

Operation

The operative technique is similar to the one described for the Binkhorst iridocapsular IOL, except that capsular flaps are redundant because the elongated inferior loop is relatively easy to place in the inferior capsular bag, and the superior loop is anchored by the clip and does not have to be in the superior bag. The incision should be the optic width plus 2.0 mm because this is a two-plane IOL. The combined diameter of the optic and haptic carrier is 6.2 mm; therefore an 8.2-mm incision is required. An ECCE section is closed to the necessary size, whereas a KPE is enlarged to 8.2 mm. The superior haptic rim of the IOL is held with Clayman forceps, and the lens is inserted into the anterior chamber under an air bubble, ideally with about a 5.0-mm pupil. The inferior loop is slid behind the iris and into the inferior capsular bag (Fig. 4-20). It should be remembered that the inferior loop is elongated, so care is taken to avoid excessive inferior IOL displacement, lest the capsule be ruptured or the zonules dialysed. The IOL is steadied with the implant forceps as the superior iris is lifted over the superior IOL loop, with either Hoskin forceps or an iris hook held in the left hand, in a maneuver similar to that shown in Fig. 4-14. After this is accomplished, the IOL is centered (Fig. 4-21),

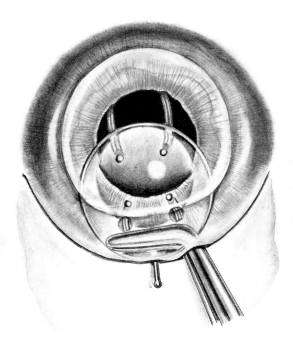

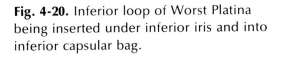

Fig. 4-20. Inferior loop of Worst Platina being inserted under inferior iris and into inferior capsular bag.

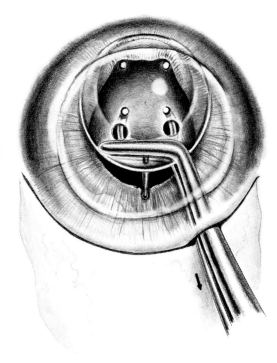

Fig. 4-21. IOL is centered with a superior motion of the holding forceps *(arrow)*.

and intracameral acetylcholine is instilled for miosis. When the miotic pupil has centered the IOL, a generous superior peripheral iridectomy is made *immediately posterior* to the platinum wire (or plastic stave). The wire must then be bent through the iridectomy and around the apex of the superior loop from back to front. This is best performed with a bimanual technique, the left hand holding an instrument to immobilize the haptic rim while the right hand bends the clip (Fig. 4-22). With the left-hand instrument, the IOL should be

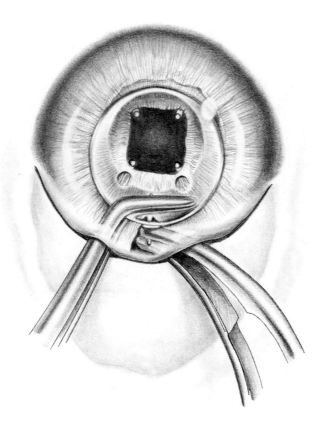

Fig. 4-22. Bending the clip with a bimanual technique.

tilted slightly anteriorly and raised superiorly to bring the superior loop into the aperture of the peripheral iridectomy. The platinum wire should be bent posteriorly with the right-hand instrument, through the aperture of the iridectomy. The wire is released and regrasped from below the apex of the superior loop; then it is bent forward around the outer aspect of the loop, thus making a reverse C-shaped clip (Fig. 4-23).

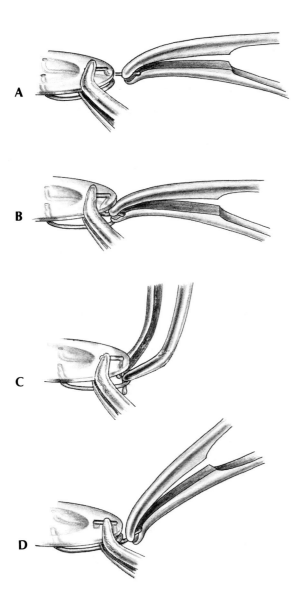

Fig. 4-23. A, The IOL raised slightly, and the stave grasped with the right-hand instrument. **B,** The stave is bent inferior and posterior. **C,** The stave is clipped so that part of it extends posteriorly at the apex of the superior loop. **D,** The tip of the stave is regrasped, drawing it around the apex of the superior loop, thus forming a clip.

Comments

A plastic stave has its own resiliency, and merely bending it posteriorly will cause it to negotiate the apex of the superior loop and then spring into position, albeit without the reverse C configuration. There are two points of special caution: first, the platinum wire is fragile and may break off with repeated manipulation. Second, if the peripheral iridectomy is too small, i.e., too peripheral, the lens will ride superiorly with the possibility of chronic dislocation of the inferior loop and/or IOL touch to the superior corneal endothelium.

There are several possibilities for other corneal endothelial damage with this IOL. First, if there is positive vitreous pressure, the clipping maneuvers are extremely difficult to perform without repeatedly collapsing the anterior chamber. Second, if the platinum clip is incompletely bent, it may protrude anteriorly and traumatize the superior corneal endothelium when the patient assumes certain positions. Third, we have previously discussed residual cortex in the superior capsular cul-de-sac (p. 126). We have seen this swell postoperatively, tilting the lens anteriorly and causing the IOL intermittently to touch the superior corneal endothelium. Last, bending the clip can be a challenging maneuver. Various instruments and techniques have been designed to facilitate the clipping, which, of itself, can result in persistent superior corneal edema.

Parenthetically, the Worst Platina clip IOL is also used after an ICCE by some surgeons, although that kind of usage is declining. All our comments on insertion still apply, along with the added risk of vitreous loss at the peripheral iridectomy as the clip is being bent. Furthermore, the peripheral iridectomy is crucial. If it is too small and peripheral, the IOL will ride superiorly as noted above; on the other hand, if the iridectomy is too large, the IOL will tend to ride low, the net effect being suspension of the IOL from the apex of the peripheral iridectomy by the clip. This can result in an undesirable pendular pseudophacodonesis during eye movement.

Worst's clip concept attempted to overcome the fixation difficulties of the Binkhorst iridocapsular IOL. Yet the clip produced its own problems both in technique and postoperatively. Some surgeons have avoided using the clip by fixating the Platina IOL with an iris suture, producing a Worst Medallion-type IOL with the loops vertical instead of horizontal. To repeat our oft-stated theme, a single-plane IOL requires no iris sutures or clips and tends to preserve a formed anterior chamber during IOL insertion. As such, the operation is easier and the opportunities for intraoperative complications less. The usage of iridocapsular IOLs has declined in the past few years with recognition of these facts.

Five

Posterior chamber intraocular lenses

GENERAL PRINCIPLES

The first intraocular lens of the modern era—a posterior chamber IOL—was inserted by Ridley in 1949. There were numerous problems with the Ridley lens, and because of them the concept of posterior chamber pseudophakia fell into disrepute until the late 1970s. Although other surgeons had reinvestigated posterior chamber IOLs, it was Shearing who introduced and popularized a viable lens, which stimulated a new interest in the topic. The dimension of this interest can be estimated by considering that in 1977 posterior chamber IOLs accounted for less than 1% of the total IOLs implanted, yet by 1981 they made up 22% of the total.

In this chapter, we primarily discuss J-loop posterior chamber lenses, as exemplified by the Shearing IOL. There are posterior chamber lenses with other types of fixation, but they have stimulated little widespread interest in the ophthalmologic profession.

With a minor exception, all of the currently available posterior chamber IOLs are inserted in conjunction with an ECCE, a heretofore relatively unfamiliar technique to many ophthalmic surgeons, who have to change from ICCE. Then why the enormous popularity of posterior chamber lens, especially J-loop lenses? The answer is that they give more gratifying results to both the patient and surgeon, short term and long term. There are several reasons for this. First, once the ECCE has been mastered, the major hurdle has been overcome; the J-loop posterior chamber lens is easy to insert because of its single-plane construction thus intraoperative IOL-related complications are minimized. Second, we unreservedly state that eyes have less inflammation after ECCE and can see better earlier. Third, the incidence of CME and retinal detachment is less after ECCE, with or without a discission. Last, the lens fixates well with minimal pseudophacodonesis, and the pupil can be dilated ad lib.

J-LOOP POSTERIOR CHAMBER LENS (SHEARING LENS)
Description

This lens varies among the various manufacturers, but generally the optic is planoconvex, with the convex surface anterior. Its diameter is 6.0 mm, and two incomplete J-shaped loops originate at opposing poles of the optic. There are two to four bore holes in the optic's periphery to facilitate intracameral manipulation. The total loop diameter is approximately 13.5 mm with the loops' apexes designed to fixate in the ciliary sulcus (Fig. 5-1). The original Shearing lens was designed with the loops horizontal to the optic (Fig. 5-2).

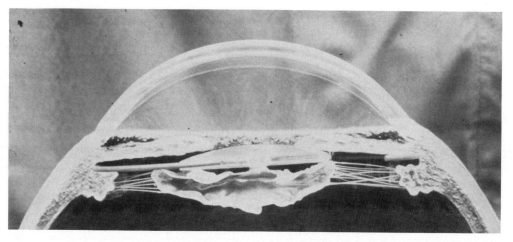

Fig. 5-1. Concept of ciliary sulcus fixation. (Courtesy Intermedics Intraocular, Inc.)

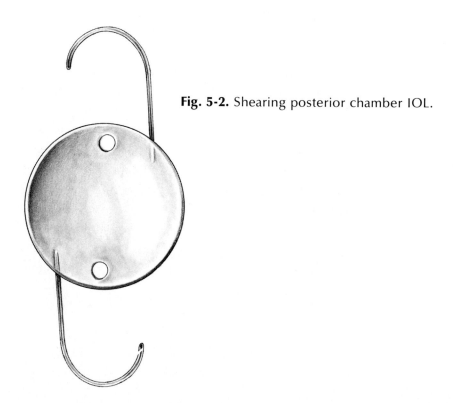

Fig. 5-2. Shearing posterior chamber IOL.

Operation

The lens is inserted after either an ECCE or a phacoemulsification. Following the techniques described in Chapter 1, in an ECCE the 12 o'clock preplaced suture in the corneal scleral section is removed. In our method of preplaced suturing, this will leave a 7.0-mm superior incision, through which the implant will be inserted. When the lens is inserted after a phacoemulsification, the initial incision is enlarged from a width of 3.0 to 7.0 mm. A right-handed surgeon would have made the initial phaco-incision at the 10:30 position. Therefore, this incision is enlarged clockwise (to the surgeon's left) so that the IOL is inserted through the customary superior section. The extent of the incision can be indicated by calipers held by an assistant or by calibrated Clayman corneal section scissors. Thereafter, the technique for insertion is identical to that following ECCE, described previously. Prior to IOL insertion, an air bubble is instilled into the anterior chamber until the iris is *slightly* concave. The superior edge of the optic is grasped with Clayman implant forceps. The optic's convex face should be anterior and the *incomplete* arm of the superior J-loop to the surgeon's right. The optic is slid into the anterior chamber without corneal retraction (Fig. 5-3), the incision being

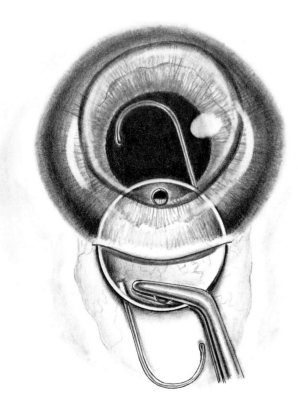

Fig. 5-3. Shearing IOL being introduced into the anterior chamber. (Shown with a 7-mm incision following a KPE.)

separated by the advancing inferior loop. The implant is slid inferiorly until the inferior J-loop is under the inferior iris and the optic is completely within the anterior chamber (Fig. 5-4). The superior cornea not infrequently bends on itself during this maneuver. This may be desirable, since it protects the superior endothelium during IOL insertion. The invagination of the superior cornea is corrected as the implant forceps are released and withdrawn from the anterior chamber. Occasionally, the whole optic cannot be placed in the anterior chamber on the initial maneuver. If the optic is released before its total diameter comes into the anterior chamber, it may pivot abruptly posteriorly as the implant forceps are released, with consequent risk of perforation of the posterior capsule from the inferior loop or optic edge. This can be obviated by *gently* releasing the forceps and sliding them slightly to the right as they are withdrawn from the optic. If part of the optic remains out of the anterior chamber, it is nudged into position with the tips of the forceps. The most common reason for inability to insert the optic is loss of the air bubble; additional aliquots of air may be reinstilled into the anterior chamber as required.

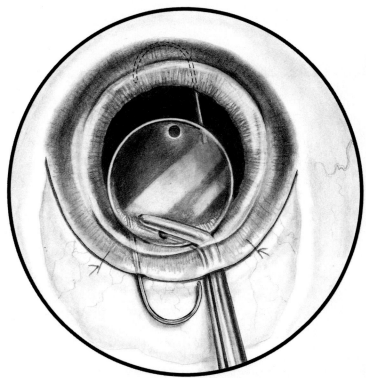

Fig. 5-4. Inferior loop slid under inferior iris. Whole optic is in anterior chamber. (Shown following an ECCE.)

What we have, then, is the optic and inferior loop in the anterior chamber and part of the superior loop extending out of the incision. In the classic Shearing technique, the tip of the incomplete arm of the superior J-loop is grasped with forceps (e.g., Kelman-McPherson forceps) (Fig. 5-5). The loop is compressed by pushing it inferiorly. This not only compresses the loop but also slides the optic and inferior loop further inferiorly. Therefore the superior loop is completely within the anterior chamber in the compressed position. The inferior motion of the IOL is continued until the apex of the superior compressed loop has cleared the pupillary margin (Fig. 5-6). At this point the loop is released from the forceps so that it springs into position posterior to the superior iris (Fig. 5-7). The Shearing technique of insertion is summarized (Fig. 5-8) and shown in sagittal view. Fig. 5-9 shows the Shearing IOL in situ.

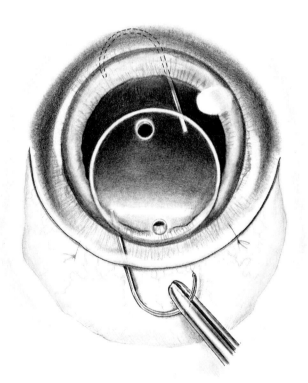

Fig. 5-5. Tip of superior loop grasped with forceps.

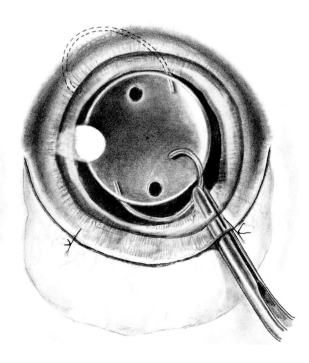

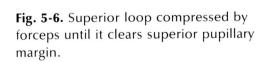

Fig. 5-6. Superior loop compressed by forceps until it clears superior pupillary margin.

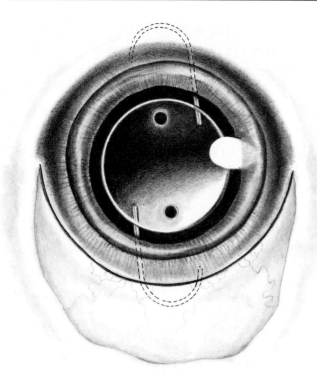

Fig. 5-7. Shearing IOL in situ.

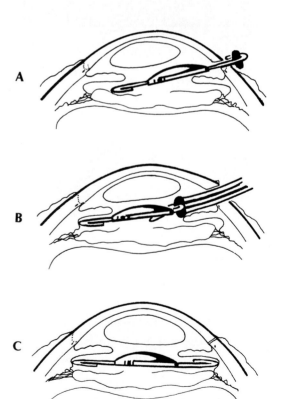

Fig. 5-8. A, Sagittal view, inferior loop inserted under inferior iris. **B,** Sagittal view, superior loop compressed until it clears pupillary margin. **C,** Sagittal view, superior loop springs into position posterior to superior iris.

Occasionally, the superior loop springs *anteriorly* to the iris and is surprisingly difficult to regrasp intracamerally. If that occurs, we hook the apex of the superior loop and draw it into the incision where it is regrasped and correctly inserted. The forceps are withdrawn from the eye, and the optic is centered with either a Jaffe hook or a Clayman guide (see Fig. 5-24, *B*). A peripheral iridectomy is performed, and the air bubble is replaced with balanced saline. A discission is performed as described in Chapter 1 and in Fig. 5-29. The section is sutured according to the surgeon's preference.

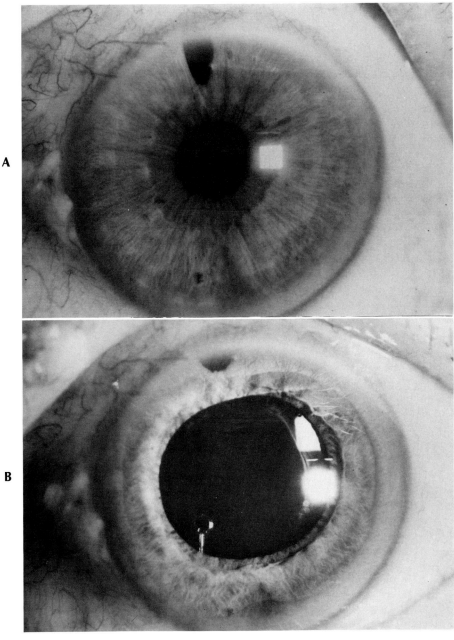

Fig. 5-9. A, Shearing IOL in situ. **B,** Shearing lens in situ with pupillary dilation. (From Jaffe, N.S.: Cataract surgery and ifs complications, ed. 3, St. Louis, 1981, The C.V. Mosby Co.

OTHER LENS DESIGNS
Kratz/Shearing modification

There have been variations on Shearing's initial design. Kratz proposed an important evolutionary step, in which the haptic loops are angulated forward (Fig. 5-10). This, in turn, displaces the optic further posteriorly and away from the pupil (Fig. 5-11) and largely obviates pupillary capture, which is discussed in Chapter 8. Briefly, *pupillary capture* refers to the condition in which the optic is "captured" by a constricting pupil so that all or part of the optic rests anteriorly to the iris while the haptic loops remain posterior to the iris in the ciliary sulcus.

The Kratz anterior loop angulation is most desirable and only fractionally affects insertion in two respects. First, as the inferior loop is inserted, instead of sliding under the inferior iris it may slide anterior because of its anterior angulation. If this is the case, the IOL should be withdrawn slightly until the inferior loop's apex is just centrad to the pupillary border and then reinserted with a lifting motion on the superior loop, which will pivot the inferior loop posteriorly so that it may then be slid behind the iris. Second, the anterior angulation may prevent the superior loop from springing into position posterior to the iris after its release from the forceps. With the angulated model IOL, the apex of the superior loop should be guided behind the iris and then released from the forceps.

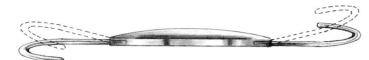

Fig. 5-10. Sagittal view of Shearing IOL showing Kratz anterior angulated loops *(broken line),* compared to original horizontal looped model.

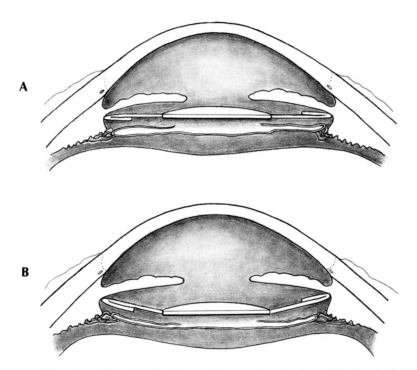

Fig. 5-11. A, Shearing IOL with horizontal loops, in situ (sagittal view). **B,** Kratz modification of Shearing IOL, in situ. Note that the optic is displaced posteriorly away from the pupil by the angulated loops.

Kratz/Sinskey lens

The loop design was further modified by both Kratz and Sinskey. The loop curvature was changed, but the forward angulation was retained. Most important, the loop origination was moved closer to the horizontal poles of the optic, which in effect increased the total length (not diameter) of loop material per lens (Fig. 5-12). This, in turn, made the loops more pliable and compressible and supposedly less likely to traumatize the inferior zonules on insertion. The technique of insertion (Fig. 5-13) is the same as noted before. The loops are more compressible and the lens is easy to insert. However, when the pupil becomes miotic, the superior loop may be difficult to insert, since there is a longer length to compress before it can clear the superior pupillary margin and be guided back to a position posterior to the iris. Fig. 5-13 shows the Kratz/Sinskey IOL in situ.

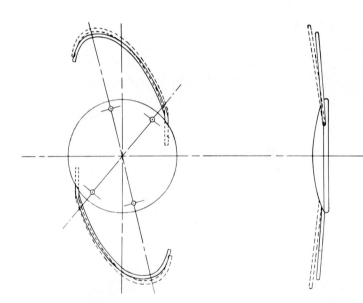

Fig. 5-12. Schematic of Kratz/Sinskey posterior chamber IOL (broken lines show optional 14-mm diameter haptic loops).

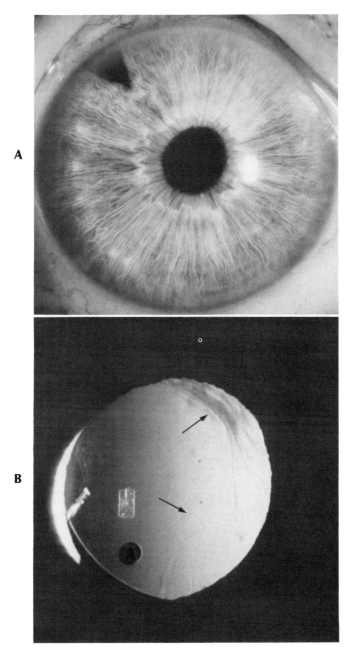

Fig. 5-13. A, Kratz/Sinskey posterior chamber IOL in situ. Since the optic and loops are posterior to the iris, the IOL is invisible in this photograph. **B,** Same patients with pupil dilated. Note margins of posterior capsulotomy *(arrows),* and optic bore hole *(A).*

Simcoe lens

Simcoe has had a long interest in J-loop posterior chamber pseudo-phakia. The Simcoe lens has an optic similar to that of the Shearing lens, but the loops differ quite radically. They are longer and more curved (Fig. 5-14). Simcoe claims that the radius of the curved loops distributes the tensile strength of the loop over a wider area and obviates trauma to the eye. He further states that the lens centers better than other J-loop models (Fig. 5-15). Currently, his loops are not angulated anteriorly.

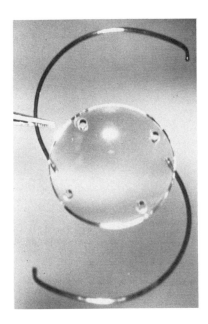

Fig. 5-14. Simcoe posterior chamber IOL.
(Courtesy Dr. C. William Simcoe.)

Fig. 5-15. Excellent centration of Simcoe IOL.
Note posterior capsulotomy *(arrows).*
(Courtesy Dr. C. William Simcoe.)

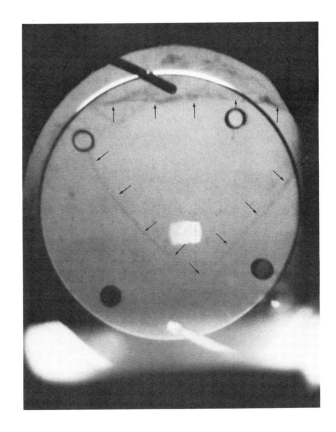

After an ECCE, the lens is inserted through a 7.0- to 8.0-mm incision (Fig. 5-16, *A*) so that the inferior loop is positioned behind the iris (Fig. 5-16, *B*). The superior loop is placed into the anterior chamber, anterior to the iris (Fig. 5-16, *C*). At this point, Simcoe advocates completely closing the section (Fig. 5-16, *D*) before "dialing" the superior loop into position with a single-instrument technique. The advancing convex edge of the superior loop mechanically distorts the pupil, permitting the loop to fall into place posterior to the iris (Fig. 5-16, *E*).

The Simcoe lens, as well as some of the other J-loop posterior chamber lenses, is available with a shorter loop diameter so that both loops can be placed within the capsular bag. Posterior chamber IOLs fixate so well that this seems to us to be an unnecessary complexity, which adds nothing to the final result.

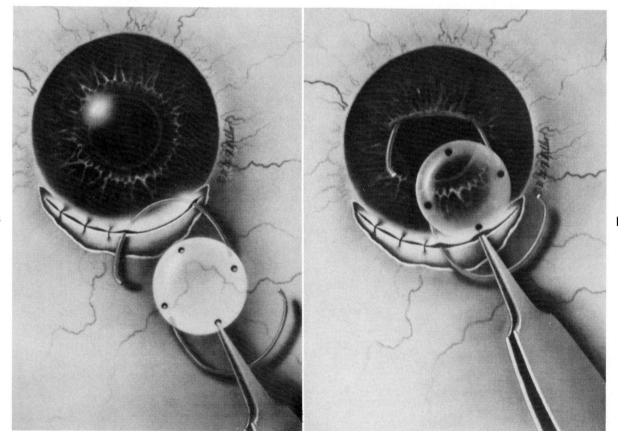

A

B

Fig. 5-16. A, Insertion of Simcoe IOL into anterior chamber. **B,** Inferior loop positioned under inferior iris. **C,** Superior foot placed into anterior chamber. **D,** Incision is closed. **E,** Superior foot "dialed" into position with a rotatory motion. (Courtesy Intermedics Intraocular, Inc.)

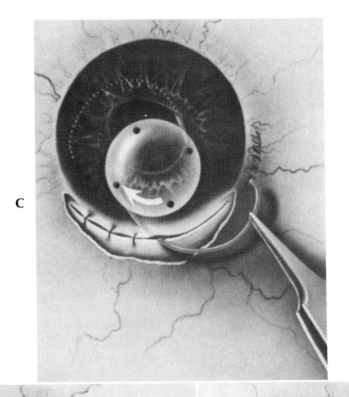

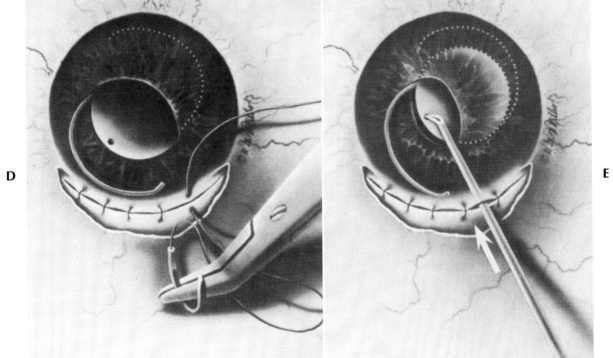

Clayman lens

The cardinal feature of the Clayman posterior chamber IOL is the 6.0-mm vertical × 5.0-mm horizontal oval optic (Fig. 5-17). In these figures the lens has Kratz/Sinskey loops with anterior angulation, but it is suitable for any J-type loop configuration. Apart from the IOL's lightness, it can be inserted through a 5.0-mm *plus* incision (Fig. 5-18). By *plus* we mean an incision fractionally greater than 5.0 mm (Fig. 5-19). The actual Clayman technique for positioning the loops is described in the following pages. The lens centers very well (Fig. 5-20) and requires less suturing to close the incision (Fig. 5-21).

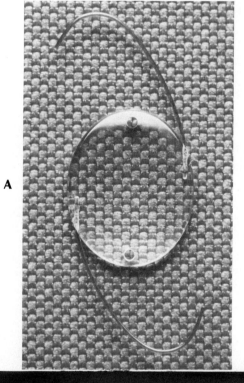

A

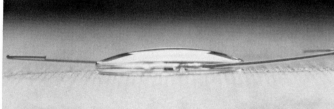

B

Fig. 5-17. A, Clayman posterior chamber IOL. Note oval optic. **B,** Clayman posterior chamber IOL (sagittal view).

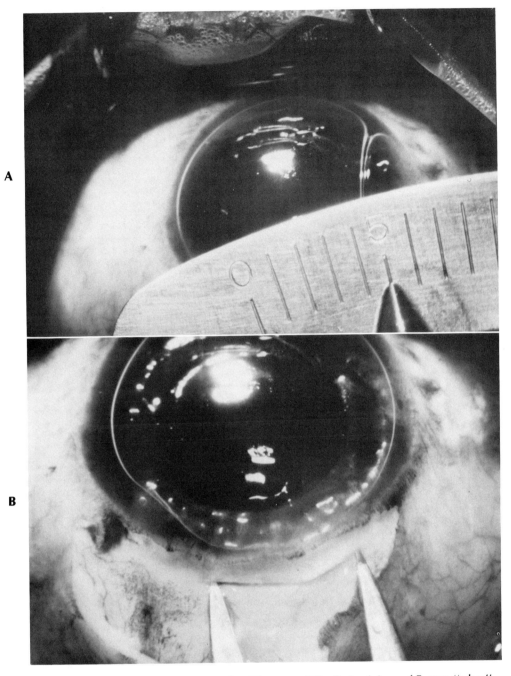

Fig. 5-18. A, Calipers set at 5 mm for Clayman IOL. **B,** Incision of 5-mm "plus" for insertion of Clayman IOL.

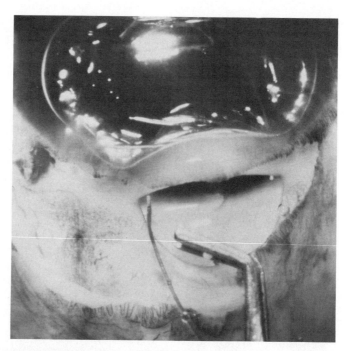

Fig. 5-19. Clayman IOL being inserted through a 5-mm "plus" incision. Note small incision helps preserve air bubble as incision is "corked" by advancing optic.

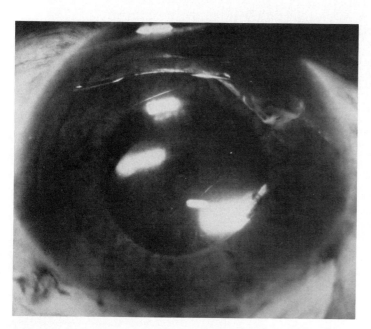

Fig. 5-20. Clayman IOL after insertion. Note centration in dilated pupil.

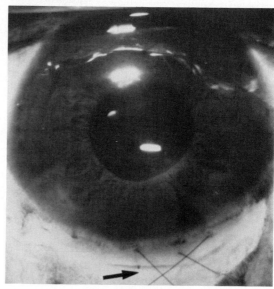

Fig. 5-21. Suture closure *(arrow)* of small incision following insertion of Clayman IOL.

MODIFICATION OF INSERTION

A correctly and securely positioned posterior chamber lens requires an intact posterior capsule prior to discission. Occasionally, a setting-sun syndrome is seen in the postoperative period with J-loop lenses (Chapter 8). In this syndrome a heretofore correctly positioned IOL sinks inferiorly so that there is an aphakic crescent superior to the optic (hence the name *setting sun*). This is presumably caused by inadvertent dialysis of the inferior zonules during insertion of the inferior loops and/or trauma to the inferior zonules during excessive inferior displacement of the IOL as attempts are made to position the superior loop. This displacement was especially likely to occur when the pupil constricted before positioning of the superior loop.

It was reasoned that, if the iris was retracted as the superior loop was being inserted, there would be less inferior movement of the IOL required; this led to the innovation of various two-handed maneuvers for IOL insertion. The further refinement of these techniques was prompted by the occasional observation of a superior loop prolapsing through the peripheral iridectomy (Fig. 5-22). If the loop was in a position remote from the iridectomy, this could not occur; thus surgeons began to rotate the IOL into a more horizontal position.

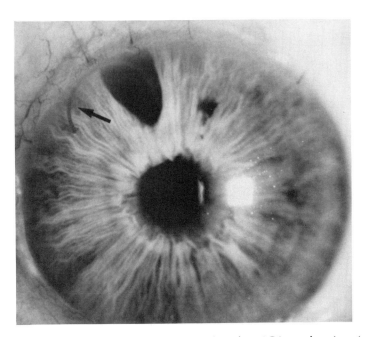

Fig. 5-22. Superior loop of J-loop posterior chamber IOL prolapsing *(arrow)* through peripheral iridectomy.

A two-handed technique of IOL insertion can simply achieve both iris retraction and IOL rotation. Several methods have been devised, and two of them are described here. The Clayman technique requires three instruments: Clayman forceps, (Fig. 5-23), and angulated iris microhook (Fig. 5-24, *A*), and an angulated lens guide (Fig. 5-24, *B*). The IOL's inferior loop is inserted under the inferior iris as already described, and preferably the whole optic is placed with Clayman forceps in the anterior chamber under an air bubble. After the forceps are withdrawn from the anterior chamber, they are used to grasp the *tip* of the superior loop. The superior loop is then placed entirely in the anterior chamber, *anterior* to the iris, with its apex in the angle imme-

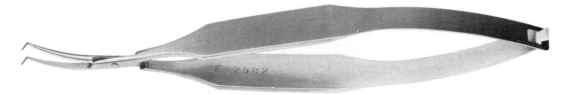

Fig. 5-23. Clayman lens implant forceps. (Courtesy Storz Instrument Company.)

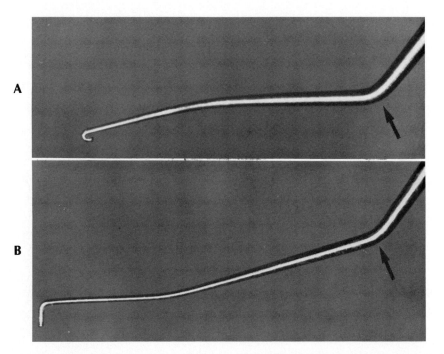

Fig. 5-24. A, Clayman angulated *(arrow)* iris microhook. **B,** Clayman angulated *(arrow)* lens guide. (From Clayman, H.M.: Am. Intra-Ocular Implant Soc. J. **6:**383, 1980.)

diately posterior to the scleral aspect of the incision. In the case of an ECCE the iris microhook is held in the surgeon's left hand and introduced into the anterior chamber at the 2 o'clock position, and the iris is retracted—all under an air bubble. In the meantime, the angulated lens guide, held in the surgeon's right hand, is slid into the anterior chamber and engages the superior bore hole of the IOL optic. The guide now "dials" the optic toward the 2 o'clock position (Fig. 5-25) so that the superior loop springs behind the re-

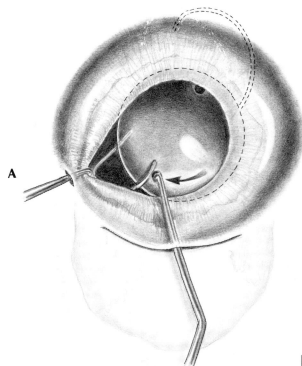

Fig. 5-25. A, Superior loop is "dialed" into position. It compresses on itself as it comes into contact with the retracted iris. **B,** Clayman lens being "dialed" into position under an air bubble, following an ECCE. Note iris retraction *(arrow)* and optic centration.

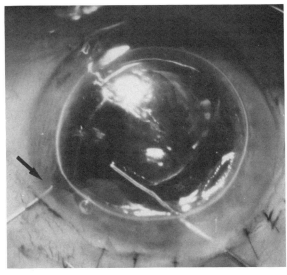

tracted iris (Fig. 5-26). The iris microhook is then released from the iris and withdrawn from the eye. The guide is used to further rotate the IOL as required, and the optic is centered, after which the guide is withdrawn (Fig. 5-27). The peripheral iridectomy is performed at the 11 o'clock position (Fig. 5-28). The posterior capsule may be left intact or a discission performed (Fig. 5-29) according to the surgeon's preference.

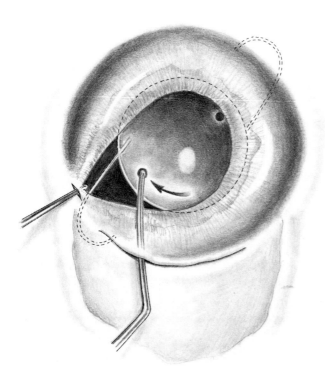

Fig. 5-26. Position of superior loop after springing behind iris. Arrow shows motion.

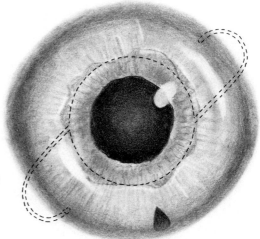

Fig. 5-27. Position of optic and loops *(broken lines)* within posterior chamber.

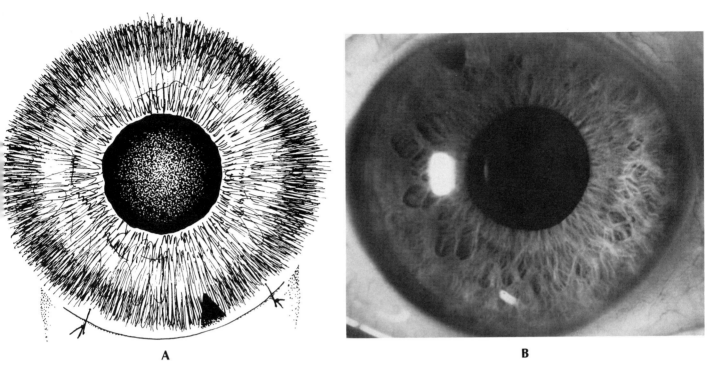

A   **B**

Fig. 5-28. A, Position of peripheral iridectomy (surgeon's view). **B,** Posterior chamber IOL in situ with peripheral iridectomy at 11 o'clock position.

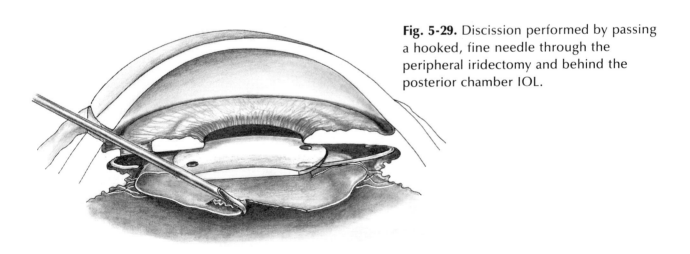

Fig. 5-29. Discission performed by passing a hooked, fine needle through the peripheral iridectomy and behind the posterior chamber IOL.

This technique works extremely well because of the mechanics involved. The angulated iris microhook is inserted through the incision, which is, of course, superior to the iris plane. When the iris is retracted, it is drawn not only peripherally but also anteriorly. The angulated lens guide imparts a posterior vector as well as a rotatory motion to the optic. Therefore, when the superior loop comes into contact with the retracted iris, it compresses itself at the apex of the retracted iris, and its posterior rotatory motion "matches" the anterior displacement of the iris. The result is that the loop springs behind the iris easily, with minimal displacement of the optic.

The IOL should be rotated only in a clockwise direction. In this direction the loops compress on themselves, shortening the overall loop diameter, and the IOL can rotate readily. If the IOL were to be rotated in the opposite direction, the loops would hyperextend, lengthening the overall loop diameter and making rotation difficult and dangerous.

In the case of a phacoemulsification, a second incision of about 1.5 mm is required at the 2 o'clock position in the limbus. Some surgeons use a two-handed KPE technique (pp. 48 and 49) and, if so, the same incision may be used for the iris microhook. If the incision has not been previously placed, it should be made prior to the enlargement of the superior section. The incision is made in the surgical limbus, just distal to clear cornea. The internal dimensions of the second incision should equal the external dimensions, lest Descemet's membrane be snagged by the iris hook. This second incision is self-sealing and needs no additional suturing.

Jaffe's technique uses Thrasher's modification of the posterior chamber IOL, in which the optic bore holes are in the 4 o'clock and 10 o'clock positions (Fig. 5-30). Jaffe inserts the lens under an air bubble with Clayman forceps, (see Fig. 5-4), placing the inferior loop under the iris at the 6 o'clock position and the whole optic into the anterior chamber, whereupon the implant forceps are released. At this point in the insertion the superior loop is still external at the incision. Simultaneously, the tip of the superior loop is grasped with Kelman-McPherson forceps held in the right hand, and the iris is retracted to the incision with an iris microhook held in the left hand (Fig. 5-31). The superior loop is gently compressed by an inferior motion made on it by the forceps held in the right hand. As the loop apex clears the edge

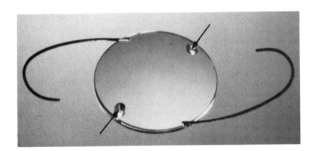

Fig. 5-30. Thrasher's modified posterior chamber IOL with bore holes *(arrows)* at 4 o'clock and 10 o'clock positions. (Courtesy Intermedics Intraocular, Inc.)

Fig. 5-31. Jaffe technique, retracting iris with the left hand and compressing superior loop with right hand.

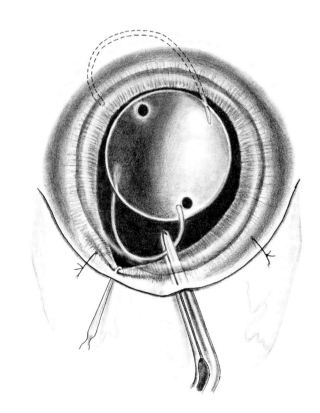

of the retracted iris, it is guided posteriorly and allowed to spring into position behind the superior iris (Fig. 5-32). The iris hook is disengaged, and both instruments are withdrawn from the anterior chamber. The IOL is then rotated with a Jaffe hook in a clockwise direction so that the loops lie in the horizontal axis (Fig. 5-35). The Jaffe hook is inserted into either the 4 o'clock or 10 o'clock bore hole, as intraoperative circumstances dictate, to effect this rotation. Thereafter, miosis is obtained, and a peripheral iridectomy and a discission are performed as noted previously.

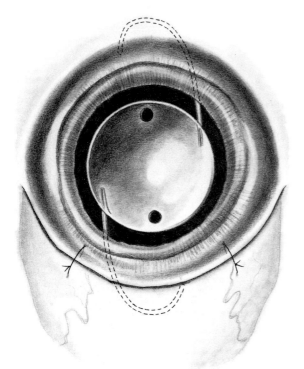

Fig. 5-32. IOL takes up position with loops posterior to iris in vertical plane.

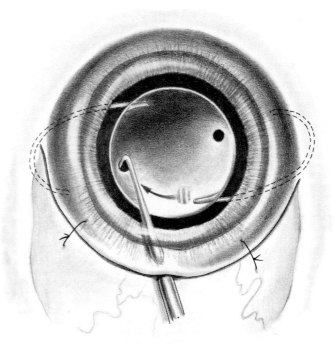

Fig. 5-33. IOL is rotated so that loops are horizontal, using a Jaffe hook.

If there is positive vitreous pressure and/or repetitive loss of the air bubble, Jaffe partially closes the incision or uses sodium hyaluronate (p. 272) before inserting the superior loop.

Irrespective of which insertion technique is used, we would like to offer a useful tip, should the pupil constrict to a diameter significantly less than that of the IOL optic. In such cases, as the inferior foot is slid under the inferior iris, try to slide at least one of the lateral edges of the optic under the corresponding iris (Fig. 5-34). This will greatly facilitate subsequent maneuvers to position the superior loop.

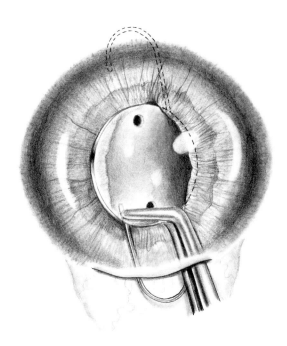

Fig. 5-34. Lateral edge of optic slid under iris to facilitate subsequent positioning of superior loop, in case where pupillary diameter is less than that of optic.

COMMENTS

There are posterior chamber IOLs in which the optic is in the posterior chamber, but the IOL has either iris or iridocapsular fixation and can therefore be used after an ICCE, ECCE, or KPE.

Severin has two iris-fixated models with the optic in the posterior chamber. Fig. 5-35 shows two vertical loops attached to the optic, both of which are positioned posteriorly to the iris. Three sets of loops are offset *anteriorly* from the optic and rest anteriorly to the iris when the IOL is in situ. In this model, Severin advocates the use of an iris-fixation suture, which is placed as described for the Binkhorst iris clip lens (p. 86). The technique of insertion is essentially the same as for the Binkhorst iris clip lens, but the two inferior anterior feet are splayed, compared with the inferior feet of the Binkhorst lens. Therefore the two-plane Severin lens lends itself poorly to closed chamber techniques.

The other model of Severin lens substitutes a polypropylene stave for the anterior superior loops (Fig. 5-36). This stave is bent through the peripheral iridectomy or iridotomy and around the apex of the posterior superior loop to form a clip. This is the same concept as that of the Worst Platina's described in Chapter 4, and the clipping technique is similar.

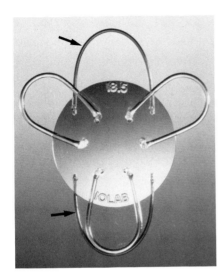

Fig. 5-35. Severin iris-fixated posterior chamber IOL. Vertical loops *(arrows)* and optic are positioned in posterior chamber. (Courtesy Iolab Corp.)

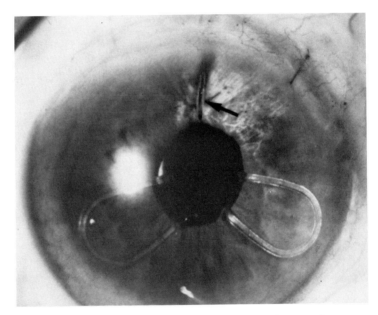

Fig. 5-36. Severin posterior chamber IOL, using a polypropylene stave *(arrow)* for fixation.

Arnott has also devised an iris or iridocapsular IOL with the optic in the posterior chamber (Fig. 5-37). The loops have a cruciate configuration quite similar to the Fyodorov-Binkhorst IOL (p. 108). The Arnott lens has had only minimal usage in the United States.

The Pearce posterior chamber lens implant is a true single-plane lens, but it is unique because an iris-fixation suture is required. The suture fixates the IOL until capsular fixation occurs, following either an ECCE or KPE. Instead of haptic loops, the lens has three solid polymethylmethacrylate feet radiating from the optic in a tripod configuration (Fig. 5-38).

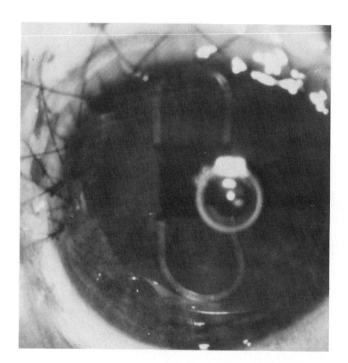

Fig. 5-37. Arnott posterior chamber IOL. (Courtesy Dr. Eric Arnott.)

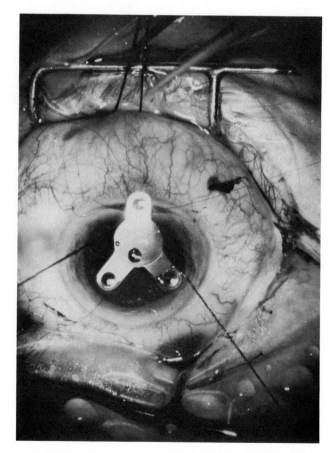

Fig. 5-38. Pearce posterior chamber IOL. (From Jaffe, N.S.: Cataract surgery and its complications, ed. 3, St. Louis, 1981, The C.V. Mosby Co.)

After the cataract extraction, a 10-0 polypropylene suture is passed through the superior iris from posterior to anterior. To do this, the needle is passed through the pupil and engages the superior iris at the 12 o'clock position, approximately 2 mm centrad to the limbus. The loose end of the suture is threaded through the hole in the superior haptic foot and tied. The free end is trimmed. Under an air bubble, the IOL's inferior feet are placed in the capsular bag, and the superior foot is positioned by retracting the iris and placing it over the foot. The slack is taken out of the fixation suture, and a small circumferential bite of anterior iris is taken, adjacent to the point where the suture emerges from the iris. A small loop is left, the long end of the suture is tied to the loop, and the knot is tightened and trimmed. The IOL is then suspended from the posterior aspect of the superior iris (Fig. 5-39). Pearce does not routinely perform either a peripheral iridectomy or a discission.

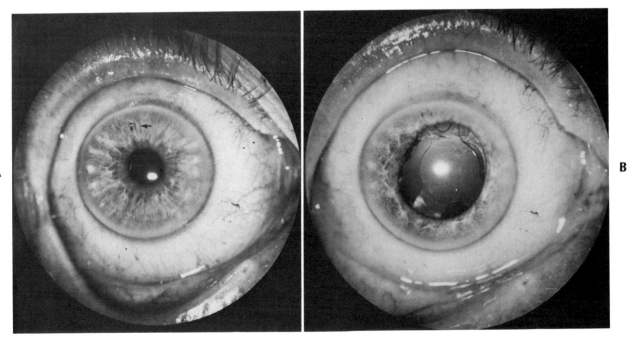

A   **B**

Fig. 5-39. A, Pearce posterior chamber IOL in situ. Note suture *(arrow).* **B,** Same eye dilated. (From Jaffe, N.S.: Cataract surgery and its complications, ed. 3, St. Louis, 1981, The C.V. Mosby Co.)

Six
Corneal complications of intraocular lenses

PREEXISTENT CORNEAL DISEASE

A frequent question that arises is whether an IOL should be inserted when corneal disease preexists with a cataract. We consider only the most common clinical entities. Certainly, an old corneal pannus would preclude neither cataract surgery nor IOL insertion (Fig. 6-1). The most common clinical problem encountered is corneal guttata, but what is its significance? Specular microscopy can be performed, but at the current state of the art a specific cell count cannot be considered as an absolute prognosticator of either corneal viability or decompensation. Cell morphology can be described, but our knowledge of the importance of aberrations in cell size and shape is incomplete. Our comments are not to deprecate specular microscopy, but rather to suggest that cell counts are not an absolute indication or contraindication for IOL surgery.

If corneal guttata exist in a solitary finding and are bilateral, we generally perform IOL surgery. However, if the guttata are unilateral and are in the cataractous eye, the surgeon must be more circumspect, because another ocular disease may be present, e.g., a pigment dispersion syndrome. When guttae occur as part of Fuchs' corneal endothelial dystrophy, the decision to operate can be very difficult. These eyes may have miotic pupils consequent to glaucoma therapy and so may require additional iris surgery (p. 197) to facilitate IOL insertion. This could produce additional endothelial trauma.

On the other hand, it could be argued that corneal-vitreous touch after an ICCE (Fig. 6-2) occurs in a high percentage of patients and may precipitate corneal decompensation in those patients with Fuchs' dystrophy. An IOL-iris diaphragm would impede the forward movement of the vitreous and preclude corneal contact. If an eye with Fuchs' dystrophy sustained corneal decompensation, would the patient's visual status be better after a pseudophakic keratoplasty than after an aphakic keratoplasty? CME is a major cause of visual loss in *both* aphakes and pseudophakes after keratoplasty, but discounting this factor, we submit that the pseudophakic eye would be superior in a unilateral case. The reason for this is the difficulty in fitting the post-keratoplasty patient with a contact lens. There are pros and cons of IOL surgery in eyes with Fuchs' dystrophy, and the patient must be involved in the decision to operate.

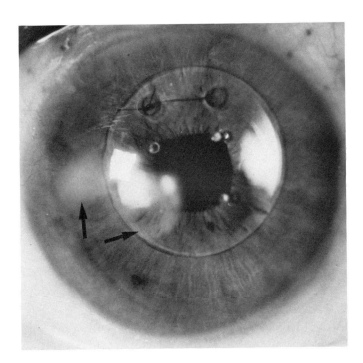

Fig. 6-1. Worst Medallion in situ in patient with preexistent corneal pannus *(arrows)*.

Fig. 6-2. Corneal-vitreous touch. Note thickened cornea *(arrow)*, secondary to contact with a large knuckle of vitreous *(V)*.

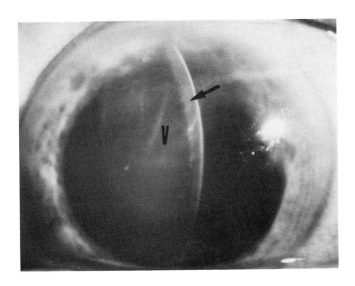

CORNEAL COMPLICATION OF IOLS

The corneal complications of IOLs are all the corneal complications of cataract surgery plus any complications induced by the insertion of the IOL and its subsequent long-term presence within the eye. Let us first consider intraoperative complications of IOL surgery.

Stripping of Descemet's membrane

A *small* tag of stripped Descemet's membrane is sometimes seen adjacent to a cataract section and is of no clinical significance; it can be avoided with careful technique. However, a detachment of more than 20% of the area of Descemet's membrane is a serious complication. There will be persistent corneal epithelial edema in the area corresponding to the detachment, and the patient will have local ocular complaints. This complication can also be the harbinger of total corneal decompensation.

The best treatment is *prevention.* A large detachment of the membrane can be caused by a cystotome, bent-tipped needle (p. 23), or other instruments; an excessively anterior incision predisposes to this complication. Care should be exercised while enlarging the incision, lest the inner (intracameral) blade of the corneal-scleral section scissors traumatize Descemet's membrane. Especially pertinent to IOLs is the size of the incision through which the lens is to be inserted. Paradoxically, closed chamber techniques have evolved to keep the anterior chamber formed and thus protect the corneal endothelium during IOL insertion. If the incision through which the IOL is inserted is too small (narrow), and especially if there is positive vitreous pressure, then there is a risk of stripping Descemet's membrane. This potential is further increased if a two-plane IOL is used, because the posterior loops, usually offset 0.5 or 0.6 mm from the optic back surface, act as a spring to push the anterior loops and/or optic anteriorly, potentiating further engagement of Descemet's membrane by the entering IOL. Collapse of the anterior chamber while instruments are within the eye also is a cause of Descemet's detachment.

Once a detachment has occurred, what is the remedy? Often this complication is not recognized at surgery, and only at a subsequent postoperative visit is that diagnosis made. If there is much detachment, it should be repaired promptly to prevent irreversible corneal changes. The detachment is invariably adjacent to the incision and usually superior. It furls posteriorly and slightly inferiorly.

To repair the detachment, place both a superior and an inferior rectus traction suture. Using a 27-gauge needle, inject a moderate aliquot of air at a convenient site in the surgical limbus (Fig. 6-3) so that the superior edge of the air bubble is bordered by the detached flap of Descemet's membrane. To facilitate this, rotate the eye upward with the inferior rectus suture and inject the air. Then *slowly* rotate the eye inferiorly with the superior rectus suture; this causes the intracameral air bubble to rise toward the incision. As this occurs, the bubble comes into contact with the Descemet's flap and unfurls it. The air bubble's continued ascent in the anterior chamber floats Descemet's membrane into its correct anatomic position, with additional air being added as required. A large detachment of Descemet's membrane requires suturing to hold it in position. Two or three interrupted 10-0 nylon sutures (Fig. 6-4) are placed in the area of the previously detached Descemet's membrane, 2.0 mm centrad to the limbus through full-thickness cornea and passed out through the scleral aspect of the surgical limbus, where they are tied and trimmed. These sutures may remain permanently, but if removal is desired, it should not be performed within 4 weeks after surgery.

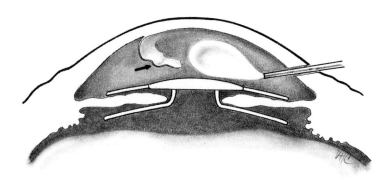

Fig. 6-3. Intracameral injection of air to unfurl a detachment of Descemet's membrane *(arrow).*

Fig. 6-4. Full-thickness corneal suturing to repair detached Descemet's membrane.

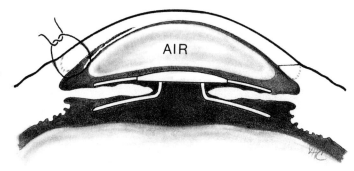

The management of a Descemet's detachment diagnosed during surgery depends on when in the operation it is noted and what type of extraction is being performed. For instance, if during an ICCE a large detachment is noted as the section is being enlarged and before cataract extraction, it is prudent to abort the operation and close the section. The detachment is then repaired with the air bubble technique described in the preceding paragraph, and the cataract removal is rescheduled for a later date. If the same detachment is noted at the conclusion of the procedure, after the IOL has been inserted, continue with the case and repair the detachment as noted previously.

The exception to this would be for those IOLs requiring a fixation suture, in which the detachment was diagnosed prior to tying the suture. The tying of the suture could conceivably entrap within it the detached Descemet's membrane, producing a situation difficult to correct technically without inducing further corneal trauma. In this contingency, the fixation suture is completely removed by cutting off the needle and sliding the suture out of the eye as expeditiously as possible. The detachment is then repaired and the patient maintained with topical miotics (p. 134) to effect IOL fixation. If necessary, a McCannel suture (p. 248) may be placed at a later date.

To momentarily digress, we have seen the corneal endothelium and presumably Descemet's membrane incorporated into the knot of an iris-fixation suture without producing a Descemet's detachment. There was, however, a Descemet's "tube" effect from the inner aspect of the cornea to the knot, without any deleterious effect.

When a detachment of Descemet's membrane is noted after any kind of cataract extraction and prior to IOL insertion, do *not* insert the IOL. The incision should be closed and the detachment repaired. The lens may be secondarily inserted at a later date (p. 283). A *small* detachment of Descemet's membrane noted at the conclusion of the procedure may be reposited with the air bubble technique without resorting to through-and-through corneal suturing. The anterior chamber should not be overfilled with air, since this can sublux the IOL posteriorly and/or contribute to pupillary block glaucoma (p. 225).

Finally, a Descemet's membrane detachment can mimic a flap of anterior capsule in an ECCE or a KPE. A small amount of irrigation fluid may show the suspicious flap to be free floating, without residual attachment, in which case it is invariably anterior capsule. If the flap is sessile and suspicious, try gently manipulating it toward the incision with a smooth spatula. If the pupil peaks at all in the direction the flap is being stroked, one is dealing with anterior capsule. This is because the anterior capsule originates at a lower level than the iris, and maneuvering the capsule toward the incision will distort the corresponding iris.

IOL-corneal touch

Corneal edema can result from intraoperative corneal endothelial damage from IOL-endothelial touch during insertion; in our discussion of surgical techniques we have stressed the importance of avoiding this (Fig. 6-5). When there is postoperative IOL-endothelial touch, there will be segmental corneal edema over the area of touch, which will eventually progress to total corneal decompensation, although that may take many months to occur (Fig. 6-6).

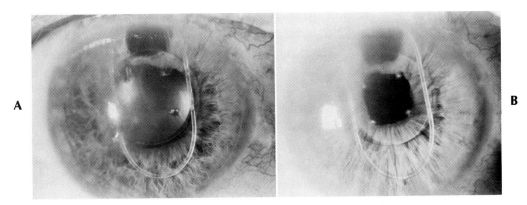

Fig. 6-5. A, Corneal edema from surgical trauma, 8 weeks postoperatively. **B,** Same eye, 6 months postoperatively. (Visual acuity—20/20.) Note residual corneal edema. (From Jaffe, N.S., and others: Pseudophakos, St. Louis, 1978, The C.V. Mosby Co.)

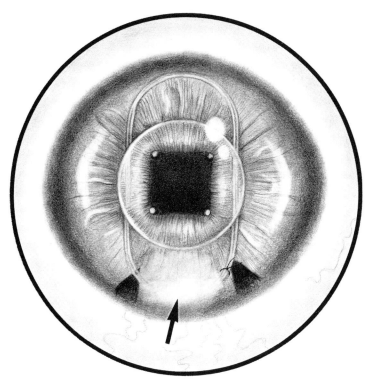

Fig. 6-6. Loop corneal endothelial touch with segmental corneal edema *(arrow).*

If the offending portion of the IOL is a haptic loop of either nylon or polypropylene, it may be amputated, leaving the IOL in situ. The loop-endothelial touch may be intermittent and dependent on the patient's position. There is a forward movement of the iris-IOL diaphragm in the prone position and this is when touch may occur (Fig. 6-7).

To amputate a loop, an incision in the limbus is made at an advantageous location. The incision should be large enough to permit the introduction of Westcott scissors, and if the anterior chamber has a propensity to collapse, sodium hyaluronate (p. 272) is used. The loop is amputated with the scissors; this involves two cuts in the loop, one at each end of the offending portion (Fig. 6-8). The amputated loop may be removed from the anterior chamber by the same Westcott scissors and closed with *gentle* pres-

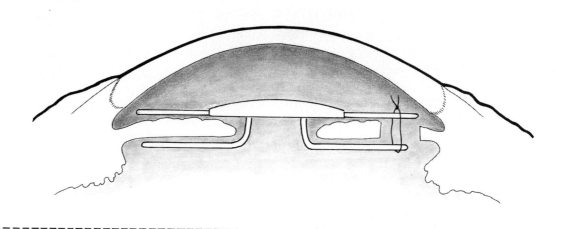

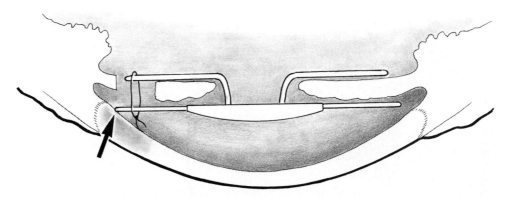

Fig. 6-7. Intermittent loop-corneal endothelial touch *(arrow)* dependent on patient position. Upper figure patient is supine; lower figure patient is prone.

sure, with the scissors acting as cross-action forceps (Fig. 6-9). If the area of loop causing the touch is secured with a fixation suture, the suture too must usually be cut prior to loop removal with either Westcott scissors or a razor knife. The severed suture is removed with Kelman-McPherson forceps. Subsequent topical miotic therapy may be indicated to fixate the IOL (p. 134). Frequently the segmental corneal edema clears after loop amputation, but on the other hand, sufficient corneal damage may have already occurred to make the changes irreversible. Such changes, compounded by the trauma of the second surgical procedure, can precipitate total corneal decompensation, which raises the question of pseudophakic keratoplasty.

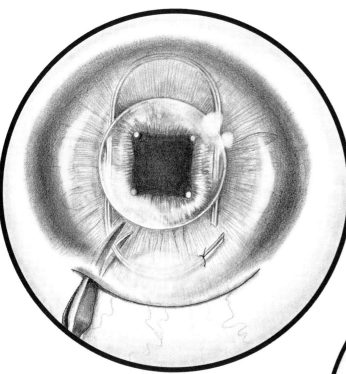

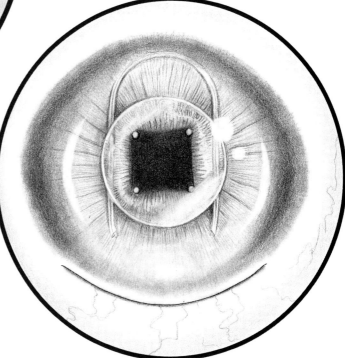

Fig. 6-8. Amputation of loop with Westcott scissors.

Fig. 6-9. Appearance of IOL after loop amputation.

Penetrating keratoplasty

The first decision to be made when a keratoplasty is planned in an eye with an IOL is whether to remove the IOL, or exchange it, or leave it in situ. A fundamental consideration is whether the corneal decompensation is part of an IOL-induced uveitis syndrome, i.e., an opaque cornea with "red" eye. If so, merely exchanging corneas will *not* rehabilitate the patient, and the IOL should be removed. In spite of a successful keratoplasty, vision is frequently compromised in these cases by chronic CME. Conversely, if the eye is quiet, i.e., an opaque cornea with a "white" eye (Fig. 6-10), the IOL may be left in situ or exchanged, as the circumstances dictate.

There is a wide variation in the techniques for keratoplasty. We will describe a technique that we find useful for most keratoplasties. For the sake of discussion, assume that the IOL is to be left in situ, and assume that the whole donor cornea is obtained with a small scleral margin. The first decision is what size donor graft goes into what size recipient bed. Generally, we will use an 8.0-mm donor graft in a 7.5-mm recipient bed (Fig. 6-11). There is good evidence that using an oversized graft reduces the incidence of postoperative ocular hypertension, and it obviously increases the area of viable endothelium in the donor.

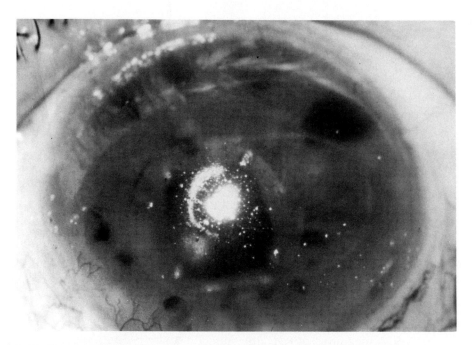

Fig. 6-10. Decompensated cornea with Binkhorst iris clip IOL in situ. (From Jaffe, N.S.: Cataract surgery and its complications, ed. 3, St. Louis, 1981, The C.V. Mosby Co.)

The Pollak punch (Storz no. E-3062) is our preferred instrument for cutting the donor corneal button. The whole donor cornea is laid, epithelial side down, on the cutting block of the punch. There is a chuck which slides within the punch, and in that chuck is placed an 8.0-mm disposable trephine. The trephine is advanced sufficiently from the chuck so that, when the punch is used, a clean-edged, full-thickness corneal button is obtained. The corneal button is punched (Fig. 6-12), and redundant margin of donor cornea and sclera is removed from around the disposable trephine. It should be noted that the circular blade of the disposable trephine has a seam in its cutting edge. Frequently, at this point, the donor button's full thickness

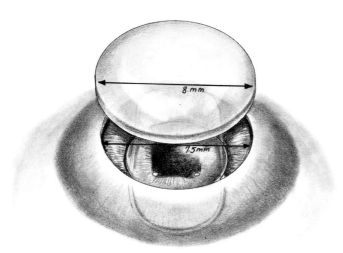

Fig. 6-11. Concept of 8.0-mm donor graft to be placed in 7.5-mm host recipient site.

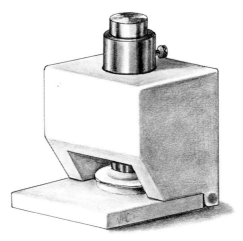

Fig. 6-12. Punching an 8.0-mm donor button with a Pollak punch.

is not cut. Therefore gently remove the redundant tissue and cut any residual attachment to the donor cornea with a razor knife. Obtain a glass Petri dish containing a gauze moistened with balanced saline. Remove the donor cornea from the trephine and place it, epithelial side down, on the moistened gauze (Fig. 6-13). The Petri dish is covered and set aside for later use. When transferring the donor cornea from the trephine to the dish, grasp the cut edge of the donor with 0.12-mm forceps over a sterile table, taking care not to drop the tissue. Occasionally the donor tissue becomes wedged in the trephine and cannot be removed with the forceps. In this case, instill a small amount of balanced saline solution in the open opposite end of the trephine. This will dislodge the tissue and make it accessible to the forceps.

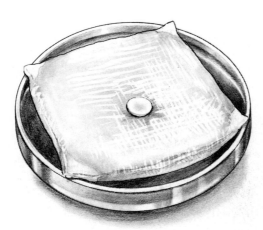

Fig. 6-13. Donor graft placed epithelial side down on moist gauze.

For the recipient eye, a 4-0 black silk superior rectus suture should be placed. A Flieringa ring is desirable and, for the average adult eye, 16.0 mm is the appropriate size. The ring is sutured to each scleral quadrant with a 6-0 black silk suture (Fig. 6-14). Under the operating microscope, mark on the patient's cornea the vertical and horizontal extremes of a 7.5-mm corneal graft. These marks are made with the tips of calipers set at 7.5 mm and are helpful in aligning the trephine under the microscope. Place and center the trephine on the patient's cornea. Then with gentle downward pressure, rotate the instrument between the thumb and forefinger, first clockwise and then counterclockwise, repetitively. As this is being performed, tip the trephine slightly to one side to cause the trephine to enter the anterior chamber in the corresponding quadrant. At this point, remove the trephine and complete the dissection of the patient's cornea with right- and left-handed corneal

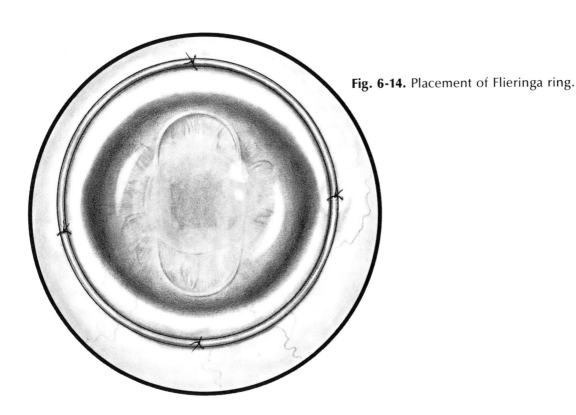

Fig. 6-14. Placement of Flieringa ring.

scissors (Fig. 6-15). The technique is to place one blade of the scissors into the anterior chamber through the perforation caused by the trephine and to cut into the circular groove produced by that instrument. After the host cornea is completely dissected, the button is passed to the scrub nurse and submitted for pathologic examination. Any shelf of tissue in the margins of the recipient corneal site should be trimmed with a razor knife. With the anterior chamber open, any manipulations of the IOL may then be performed. These may include repositioning, suture fixation, loop amputation, and even exchange. Other intraocular procedures can be done at this point, such as additional peripheral iridectomies, an anterior vitrectomy, and possibly a discission, although we prefer performing the latter with a closed chamber technique.

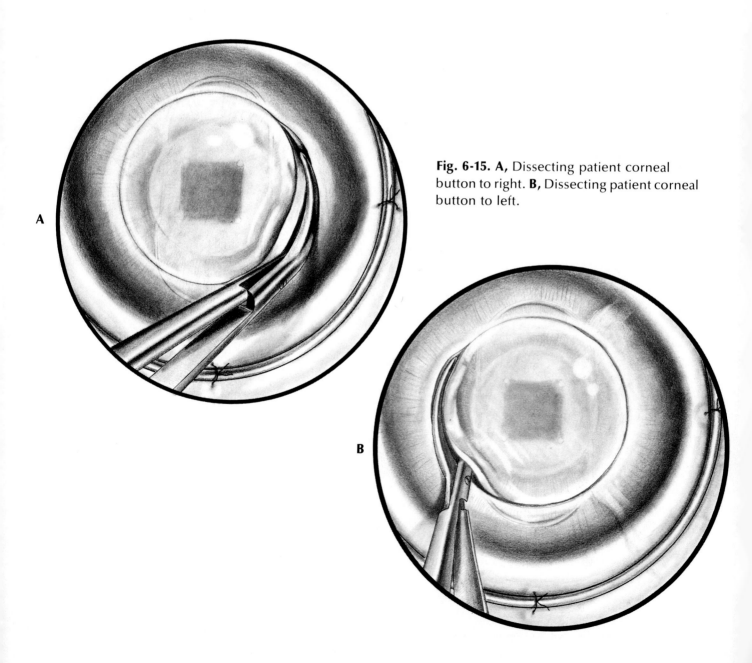

Fig. 6-15. A, Dissecting patient corneal button to right. **B,** Dissecting patient corneal button to left.

The Petri dish containing the donor tissue is opened, and the surgeon places the donor cornea in the graft site. The cornea is steadied with fine-toothed forceps (0.12 mm) held in the left hand, while a 10-0 nylon suture is passed through the margin of the donor cornea and through the recipient cornea at the 12 o'clock position, where it is tied and trimmed (Fig. 6-16). This maneuver is repeated at the 6 o'clock position, at which position the suture must be passed backhand. Additional sutures are placed at the 3 o'clock and 9 o'clock positions. The surgeon then can decide whether four additional sutures should be placed in each quadrant between the four interrupted sutures, making a total of eight sutures, or whether to proceed with the running suture.

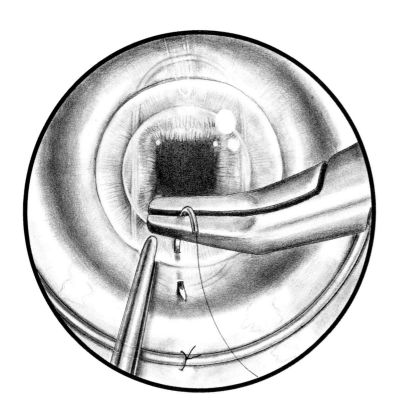

Fig. 6-16. Placement of initial 10-0 nylon suture in donor graft.

Influencing this decision would be surgeon preference and the behavior of the anterior chamber. If the chamber is formed and readily holds an air bubble, four interrupted sutures will suffice. However, with positive vitreous pressure and repeated shallowing of the anterior chamber, additional interrupted sutures should be placed to help maintain a formed anterior chamber and so prevent contact between the IOL and the donor corneal endothelium. Sodium hyaluronate (p. 272) can be very helpful in pseudophakic keratoplasties. A bolus can be placed in the anterior chamber before placing the donor cornea in the graft site (Fig. 6-17). The donor cornea will now float on a cushion of sodium hyaluronate as it is being sutured (Fig. 6-18). Moreover, the sodium hyaluronate coats the IOL, which further protects the donor corneal endothelium against potential damage from contact with the IOL.

For the running suture, approximately 6 inches is required for comfortably suturing around a 7.5-mm graft site. Therefore a 6-inch suture may be used or the second half of a 12-inch suture, the first portion having been used for the interrupted sutures. We begin running the suture at the 10 o'clock position, passing the needle through donor cornea and out through the recipient cornea, taking three or four suture bites per quadrant and proceeding clockwise. As the suture is being run, the right-handed surgeon will find it comfortable to change to backhand suturing at approximately the 4 o'clock bite and to revert to forehand suturing at the 9 o'clock bite. Each suture bite should be deep, in at least two thirds the thickness of the donor cornea and recipient tissue. When the suture has been run completely around the graft and has returned close to its point of origin, it is tightened, tied, and trimmed.

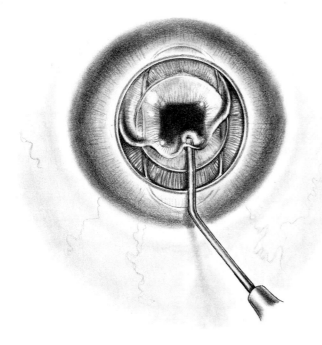

Fig. 6-17. Bolus of sodium hyaluronate instilled into the anterior chamber.

To tighten the suture, grasp the free end (i.e., the end without the needle) with tying forceps held in the right hand, to prevent the suture from being drawn into the suture tract. Hold the free end securely and with slight tension, as the running suture is progressively tightened in a clockwise direction by tying forceps held in the left hand. Next, tie the suture with three overhand ties on the first throw, squared with two individual overhand ties. Trim the suture but not at the knot; it is safer to leave ends of about 1.0 mm. When the knot has been tied, the resultant arm of the running suture bridges the incision because it originated in the donor cornea and terminated in recipient tissue. Thus, when the two ends are joined in a knot, the running suture is completed (Fig. 6-19).

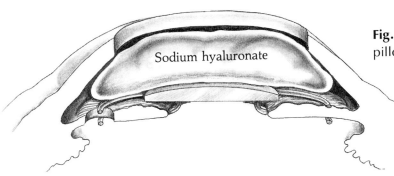

Fig. 6-18. Depiction of sodium hyaluronate's pillow effect (sagittal view).

Fig. 6-19. Appearance of pseudophakic penetrating keratoplasty, sutured with four interrupted and one running 10-0 nylon sutures.

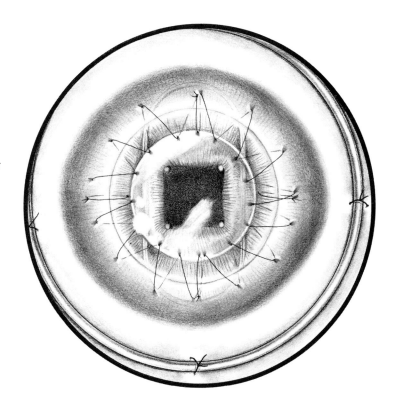

There are numerous variations in suture techniques, which include running sutures, interrupted sutures, double running sutures, or a combination. For example, some surgeons bury knots, and others remove all interrupted sutures after the running is placed. Yet another technique is to place a second running suture of 16-0 nylon (Ethicon D 4860) after removal of the interrupted sutures. The strategy here is to remove the 10-0 running suture 2 months postoperatively, leaving, the 16-0 suture in situ indefinitely.

After suturing is completed, the anterior chamber should be formed to normal psuedophakic depth by instilling balanced saline solution as required through a fine cannula inserted between donor and recipient tissue. Do not overinflate the anterior chamber, lest the IOL dislocate posteriorly. The postoperative care is the same as for a keratoplasty without an implant, topical corticosteroids being the primary treatment.

Pseudophakic corneal grafts generally do well as long as the IOL is not defective in some way. There is circumstantial evidence that an IOL exposed to the *internal* environment of the eye undergoes modification of its surface properties, and this may be beneficial to the donor endothelium when the IOL is left in situ. Fig. 6-20 shows a patient who had bilateral penetrating keratoplasties performed, having originally been operated on with ICCEs and the bilateral insertion of Worst Medallion IOLs.

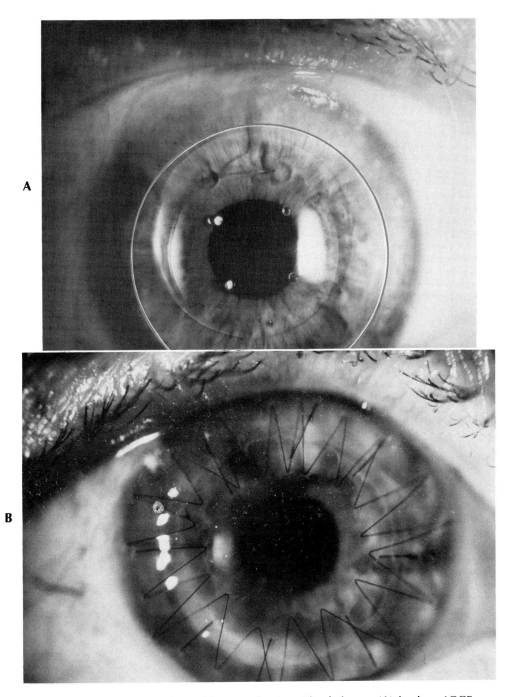

Fig. 6-20. Patient with bilateral keratoplasties. The left eye **(A)** had an ICCE with a Worst Medallion on July 12, 1977, and required a keratoplasty on March 1, 1979 (photograph retouched to show margins of graft). The right eye **(B)** had an ICCE with a Worst Medallion on June 12, 1976, and required a keratoplasty on November 9, 1981. (Visual acuity: right eye, 20/40; left eye, 20/20.)

Seven

Iris complications of intraocular lens implants

The iris complications of IOL surgery are especially significant for iris-fixated IOLs.

IRIDODIALYSIS

This can occur during enlargement of the corneal-scleral incision (Fig. 7-1) or during introduction of the lens implant into the eye. A small iridodialysis may be left alone, since it represents little more than a peripheral iridectomy. A large iridodialysis may result in a very small pupil and may also cause diplopia and other abnormal optical phenomena. In extreme cases, the pupil may not align with the optic of a posterior chamber or anterior chamber IOL. The loop of a posterior chamber IOL or the foot of an anterior chamber IOL may prolapse through the iridodialysis. Furthermore, an iris with a significant iridodialysis has an accentuated iridodonesis. If an iris-fixated IOL is then inserted, there will be an excessive pseudophacodonesis with possible corneal touch in certain patient positions (see Fig. 6-7). We suspect that these cases have also a higher incidence of CME, especially after an ICCE. A large iridodialysis should be repaired, but it is better prevented by meticulous attention to surgical technique.

The repair of a large iridodialysis requires a variation of the McCannel method (p. 248). One or two sutures are used, depending on the size of the iridodialysis. A limbal stab wound is made. With a 9-0 or 10-0 polypropylene suture attached to a cutting edge needle held backhand, a small bite is taken at the inner edge of the scleral border of the wound. The needle continues into the eye and engages the posterior border of the iris at the margin of the iridodialysis. The needle passes anteriorly through the iris and cornea (Fig. 7-2). The needle is cut from the suture, leaving approximately 4 inches of suture protruding from the cornea. The suture between the iris and cornea

190

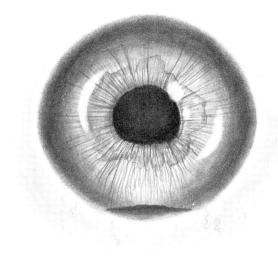

Fig. 7-1. Iridodialysis.

Fig. 7-2. McCannel suture technique for repairing iridodialysis. Suture passed through scleral margin of incision and out through cornea.

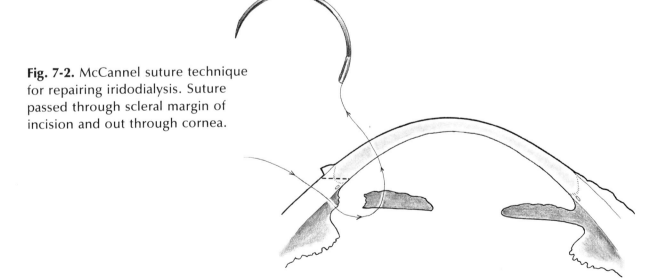

is grasped through the stab wound with an iris hook (Fig. 7-3) and drawn back through the cornea and out of the eye (Fig. 7-4). This arm of the suture is tied to the trailing arm of the suture at the bite taken through the stab wound margin (Fig. 7-5).

An alternate method is to make a larger corneal-scleral incision and draw the border of the dialyzed iris to the wound (Fig. 7-6). The iris border is then sutured (Fig. 7-7) to the inner edge of the posterior margin of the wound (Fig. 7-8).

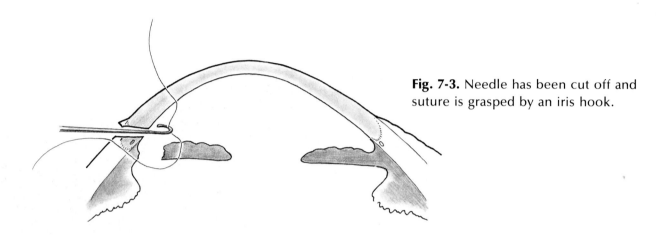

Fig. 7-3. Needle has been cut off and suture is grasped by an iris hook.

Fig. 7-4. Suture is drawn back through the cornea and out of the incision.

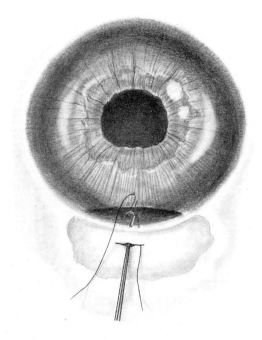

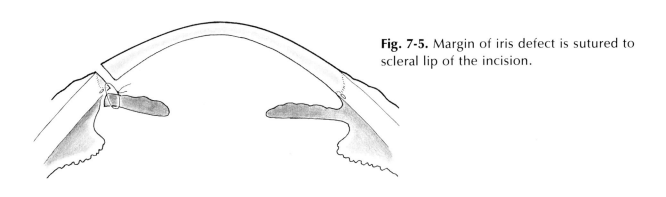

Fig. 7-5. Margin of iris defect is sutured to scleral lip of the incision.

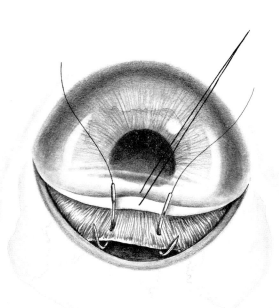

Fig. 7-6. With larger corneal-scleral incision, iris is drawn toward the incision with one or two sutures.

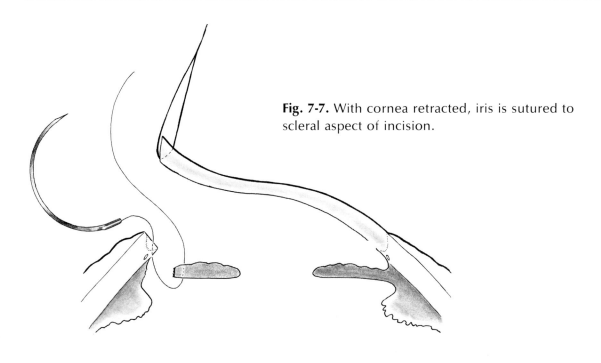

Fig. 7-7. With cornea retracted, iris is sutured to scleral aspect of incision.

Fig. 7-8. Appearance of repaired iridodialysis.

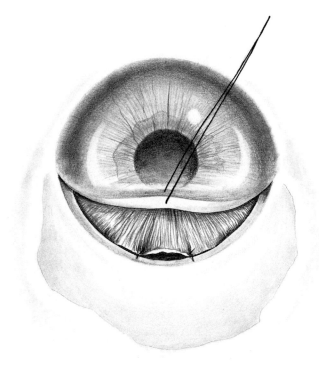

Fig. 7-9 shows a serious iridodialysis, which occurred after the iris-fixation suture around the superior loop of a Binkhorst iris clip IOL had been tied but not trimmed. The long ends of the suture were accidentally "snatched," avulsing the temporal iris root. The IOL was displaced supero-nasally and the superior loop was touching the corneal endothelium with resultant corneal edema (p. 177). In the area of the iridodialysis, the anterior hyaloid face was intact. Neither of the methods for iridodialysis repair previously described would have been suitable in this contingency, for fear of losing vitreous. Repair was effected through a trabeculectomy flap. Sodium hyaluronate was injected into the anterior chamber at this site, a hook fashioned from a 27-gauge needle (p. 23) was passed through the bolus of sodium hyaluronate, and the dialyzed iris margin was engaged (Fig. 7-10). The iris was then drawn into the trabeculectomy site and sutured to the sclera with a 10-0 polypropylene suture (Fig. 7-11). The maneuver pulled the IOL away from the corneal endothelium, but the lens was inherently unstable with marked pseudophacodonesis. The long-term ocular prognosis in such a situation is probably poor.

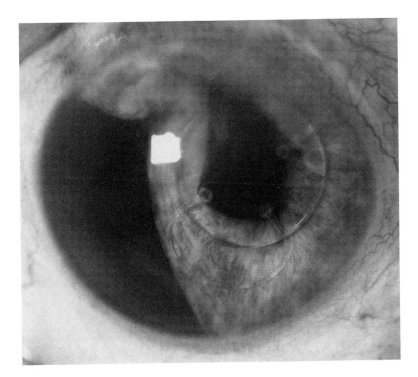

Fig. 7-9. Large iridodialysis from inadvertent snagging of IOL fixation suture.

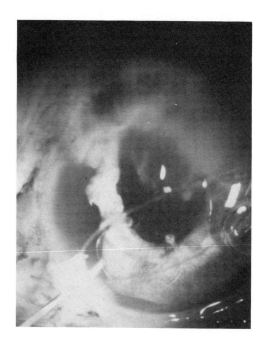

Fig. 7-10. Dialyzed iris being engaged with a hooked needle through a bolus of sodium hyaluronate.

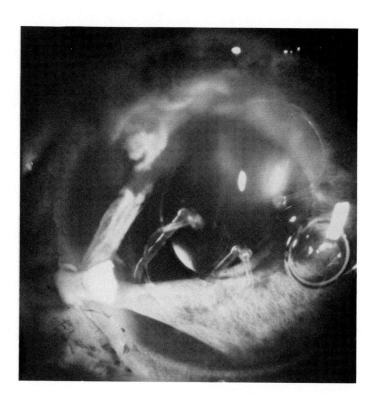

Fig. 7-11. Dialyzed iris drawn into trabeculectomy site.

MIOSIS

Inadequate pupillary dilatation may be caused by long-term miotic therapy, previous glaucoma surgery, posterior synechiae, or senile iris sphincter rigidity. Failure to administer preoperative mydriatic drops and intraoperative iris irritation both result in a small pupil also. Attempts to deliver a cataract (intracapsular) or a nucleus (extracapsular) through a small pupil may result, because of multiple iris sphincter ruptures, in a dilated atonic pupil; the attempts also increase the risk of vitreous loss. The surgical significance of the miotic pupil can be summarized by stating that the pupil must be big enough to extract the cataract safely but small enough to center and fixate an iris-fixated lens.

In an ECCE, it is impossible to perform an adequate anterior capsulectomy through a small pupil. The corneal-scleral incision is made slightly larger than usual. The iris is incised through the sphincter as will be described. Sodium hyaluronate is instilled into the anterior chamber, dilating the pupil widely and providing a deep anterior chamber for the anterior capsulectomy. The polypropylene suture is passed through the margins of the incised iris and drawn out of the eye as described in the following paragraph. The nucleus is then removed according to the surgeon's preference. The incision is temporarily closed to permit closed chamber irrigation and aspiration of residual cortical material. The wound is opened wide enough to allow the surgeon to tie and cut the suture. Lens implantation then proceeds in the usual manner. When pupillary miosis (Fig. 7-12) precludes a KPE, the prudent surgeon should convert to an ECCE and use the iridoplasty described before, if required. We qualify this because, if miosis has occurred after the anterior capsulectomy and removal of the nucleus, an iridoplasty is generally not required. The I/A, implant insertion, and discission are usually manageable through a relatively small pupil.

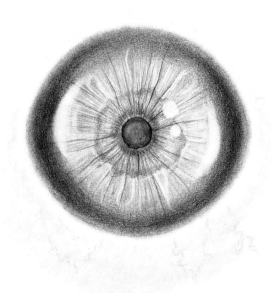

Fig. 7-12. Miotic pupil.

An iridoplasty is performed as follows. In an ICCE the usual corneal-scleral incision is made. A small peripheral iridectomy or iridotomy is made at the 12 o'clock position (Fig. 7-13). The iris is then incised with microscissors from the iridectomy through the iris sphincter (Fig. 7-14). This opens the pupil wide (Fig. 7-15). A 10-0 polypropylene suture attached to a noncutting edge needle (Ethicon no. 2794) is passed through both margins of the incised iris just above the sphincter. The suture is looped out of the eye (Fig. 7-16, *A*). After the lens is extracted, the suture is tied and cut (Fig. 7-16, *B*).

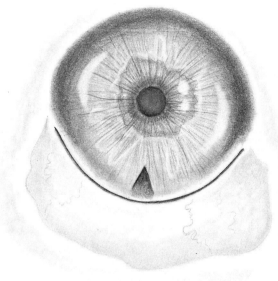

Fig. 7-13. Iridectomy at 12 o'clock position.

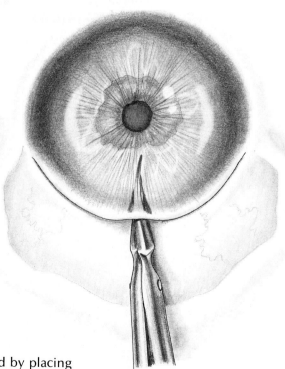

Fig. 7-14. Radial iridotomy is performed by placing one blade of scissors through aperture of peripheral iridectomy.

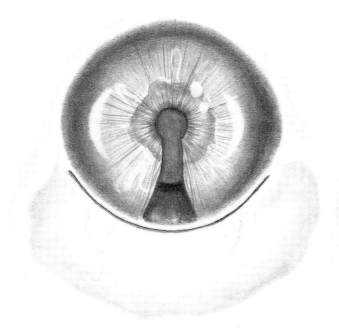

Fig. 7-15. Resultant pupillary aperture after radial iridotomy.

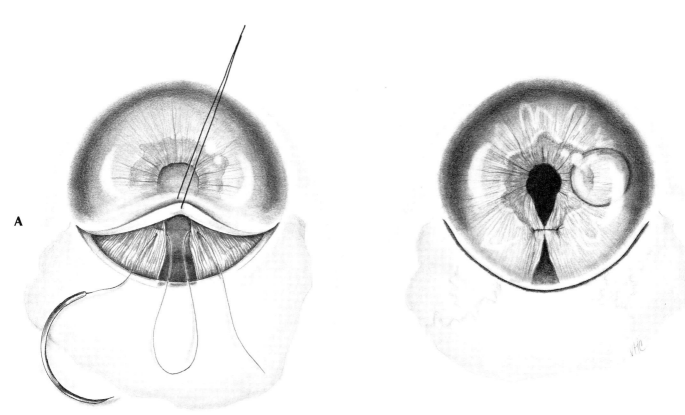

A

B

Fig. 7-16. A, Polypropylene suture passed through margins of surgical coloboma and looped out of eye. **B,** Appearance of pupil after surgical coloboma repaired.

The resultant pupil will usually have a superior notch (Fig. 7-17). The reason for this is that the iris is resutured just *above* the sphincter, not at the sphincter. The pupil was initially too small, and if it is resutured to the same size, the iris suture will cut through the iris during the insertion of an iris-fixated IOL. This would not be a consideration with other types of IOLs. The ends of the iris suture may be left long (Fig. 7-18) and threaded around the anterior superior loop of a Binkhorst iris clip lens (Fig. 7-19), thus forming the IOL fixation suture (p. 88). If the pupil is not excessively large, an iris-fixation suture is often not required with a Binkhorst iris clip lens, because the iridoplasty suture limits mydriasis, and the 4-loop design provides stability against anterior and posterior dislocation.

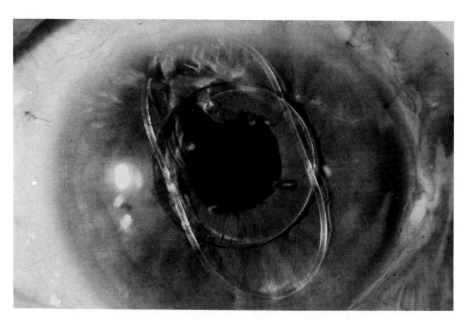

Fig. 7-17. Binkhorst 4-loop lens in situ after an iridoplasty. Note superior pupillary notch. (From Jaffe, N.S.: Cataract surgery and its complications, ed. 3, St. Louis, 1981, The C.V. Mosby Co.)

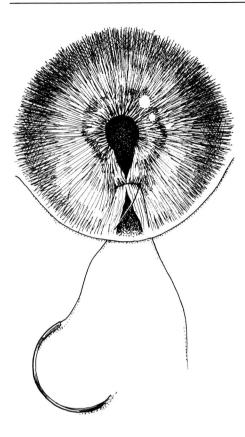

Fig. 7-18. Radial iridotomy is closed, and suture ends are left long to be subsequently threaded through anterior superior loop of IOL.

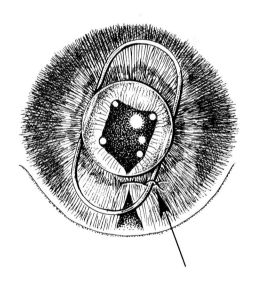

Fig. 7-19. Fixation suture *(arrow)* formed from long ends of suture used to close surgical coloboma.

A different iridoplasty technique is utilized in conjunction with the implantation of a Worst Medallion IOL. A generous corneal-scleral incision is performed. The cornea is retracted, and the iris is incised by the scissors entering through the pupil and pointing superiorly (Fig. 7-20). The incision is over just half the iris width (Fig. 7-21). The resultant pupil is shaped like

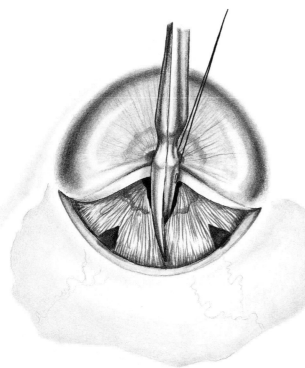

Fig. 7-20. Radial iridotomy performed with scissors entering through pupil.

Fig. 7-21. Extent of radial iridotomy *(broken lines)*.

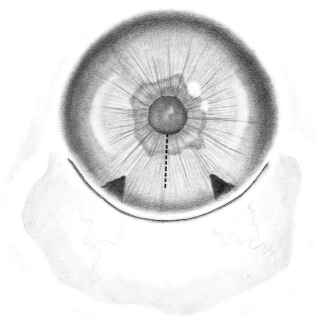

an upside-down ice cream cone, with the apex of the cone pointing to the 12 o'clock position (Fig. 7-22). A 9-0 polypropylene suture is passed through the margins of the surgical coloboma and looped out of the eye (Fig. 7-23). The cataract is removed by either an ICCE or ECCE according to the surgeon's preference. The iris suture is tied, *retaining the needle on the suture* and leaving

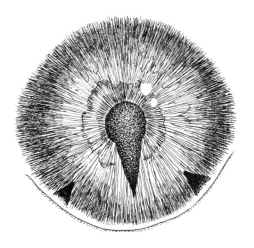

Fig. 7-22. Ice cream cone appearance of pupil after radial iridotomy.

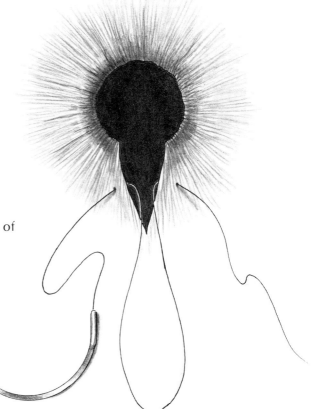

Fig. 7-23. Suture is placed through margins of surgical coloboma and looped out of eye.

the suture ends long (Fig. 7-24). This suture is then threaded through the holes of the Worst Medallion IOL as previously described (see Fig. 3-25), and the IOL is inserted (Fig. 7-25). The suture is tied and trimmed (see Fig. 3-32), and the IOL is centered as required (Fig. 7-26). Fig. 7-27 shows a patient who had this type of iridoplasty, with a Worst Medallion IOL in situ.

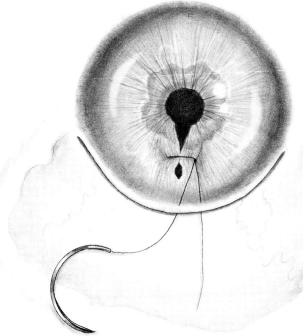

Fig. 7-24. Suture tied; needle is left on for subsequent threading through holes in IOL.

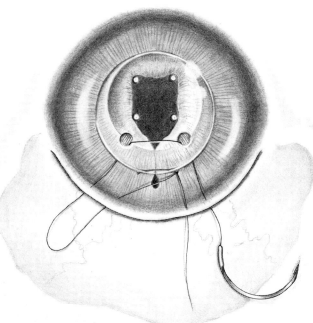

Fig. 7-25. Worst Medallion is inserted utilizing coloboma repair suture as fixation suture.

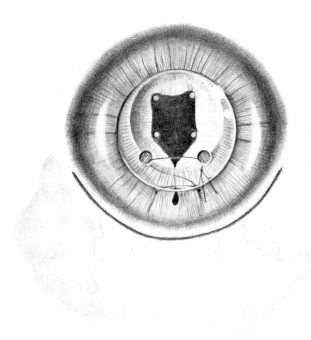

Fig. 7-26. Appearance of eye after coloboma has been repaired and fixation suture has been tied and trimmed.

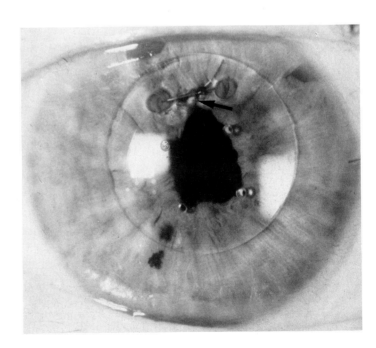

Fig. 7-27. Worst Medallion in situ after iridoplasty repair *(arrow)*.

Surgical techniques restoring iris integrity are essential only for iris-fixated lenses. As stated in Chapter 2, an anterior chamber IOL may be used to bridge an iris defect, and an intact iris is not required for posterior chamber lens fixation (with the exception of the Severin- and Arnott-type IOLs discussed on pp. 168 to 170).

Fig. 7-28, *A* shows a patient with a Shearing-type IOL in situ who had multiple sphincterotomies prior to cataract extraction. The lens fixation does not require the pupil to be re-formed (Fig. 7-28, *B*). The patient had been receiving chronic miotic therapy; Fig. 7-28, *C*, shows the maximum dilatation of the fellow eye.

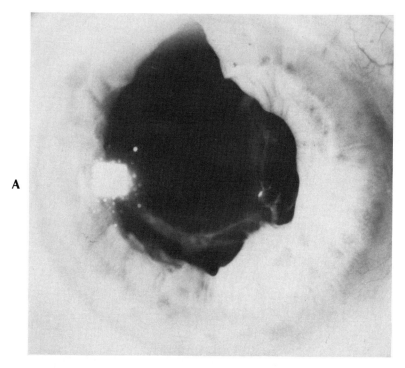

A

Fig. 7-28. A, Shearing-type IOL in situ in an eye with multiple sphincterotomies. **B,** Same eye, transilluminated. Note IOL fixation is independent of iris integrity. **C,** Fellow eye showing maximum dilatation.

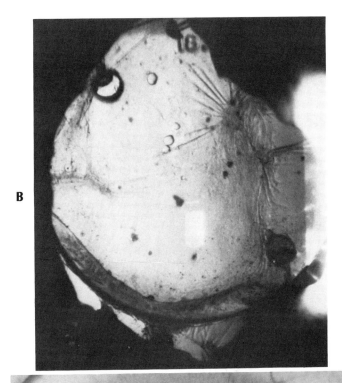

B

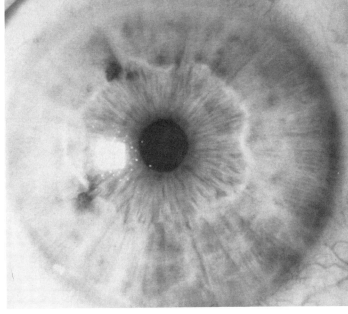

C

The technique for performing multiple sphincterotomies involves the use of microscissors (e.g., Vannas scissors) through a small incision (Fig. 7-29). This procedure should be performed under an air bubble or with the aid of sodium hyaluronate. The resultant pupil is shown in Fig. 7-30.

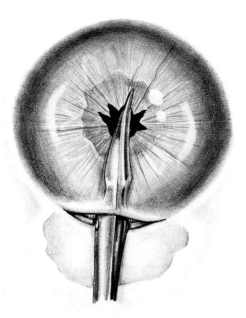

Fig. 7-29. Technique for performing multiple sphincterotomies.

Fig. 7-30. Appearance of pupil after multiple sphincterotomies.

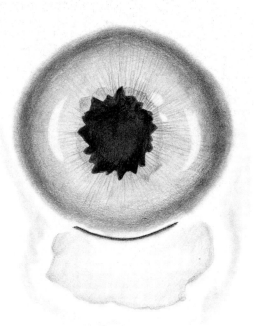

MYDRIASIS

An eye may exhibit mydriasis for a variety of reasons. The most common example encountered by the cataract surgeon is the eye that has sustained a previous attack of acute glaucoma, resulting in a pupil of about 7.0 mm, which is peaked superiorly with areas of iris atrophy. Again let us state that an iris-fixated IOL requires a viable iris and a secure iris sphincter for fixation and centration, and a mydriatic pupil requires repair when this type of IOL is to be inserted (Fig. 7-31). In other types of IOL, repair of the mydriatic pupil is not mandatory but may be desirable for cosmetic reasons. In an intracapsular case, a 10-0 polypropylene suture is passed through the iris sphincter at the 10:30 position, regrasped, and then passed through the iris at the 2 o'clock position. The suture is looped out of the eye, and the cataract is extracted. The suture is tightened and tied, which reduces the diameter of the pupil. The suture ends can be left long and threaded through the implant as previously described, thus providing a fixation suture. When an ECCE is performed, the suture can be placed either before or after cataract extraction, provided that the posterior capsule is intact. With a KPE, the suture is passed after cataract extraction, after the insertion has been sufficiently enlarged to permit IOL insertion. This enlarged incision is also required to

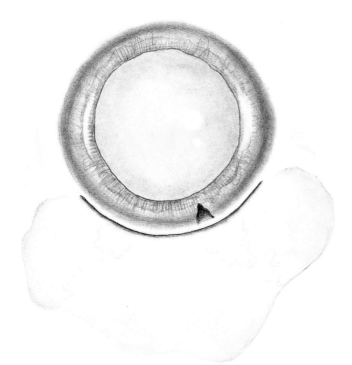

Fig. 7-31. Mydriatic pupil with previous peripheral iridectomy.

pass the iris suture safely. In Fig. 7-32, a Shearing-type IOL has been inserted into an eye with excess mydriasis. The lens loop is rotated away from the peripheral iridectomy (see Fig. 5-22), and a 10-0 polypropylene suture is placed through the iris at the 10 and 2 o'clock positions (Fig. 7-33). The suture is tied, reducing the pupil diameter (Fig. 7-34). An eye with a Shearing-type lens in situ and a sutured iris is shown in Fig. 7-35.

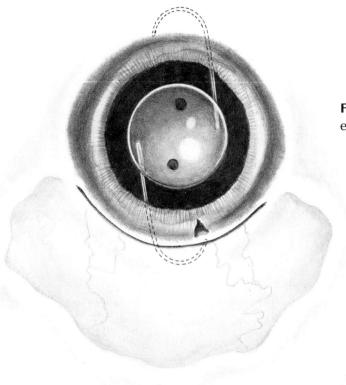

Fig. 7-32. Insertion of a Shearing-type IOL into eye with excess mydriasis.

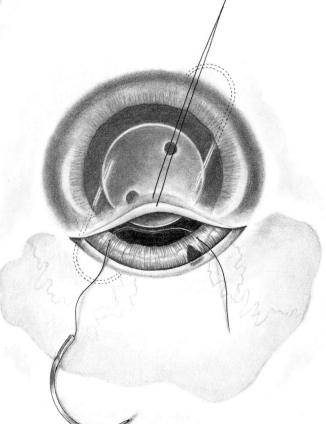

Fig. 7-33. Lens loop rotated away from peripheral iridectomy. Suture passed through iris.

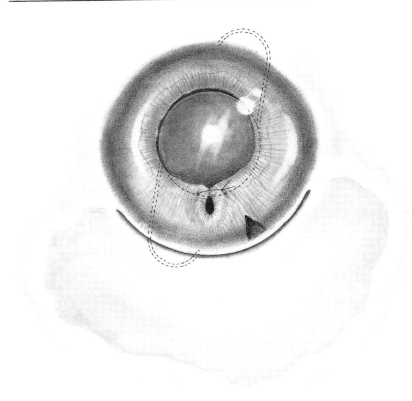

Fig. 7-34. Mydriatic pupil sutured, reducing diameter of pupil.

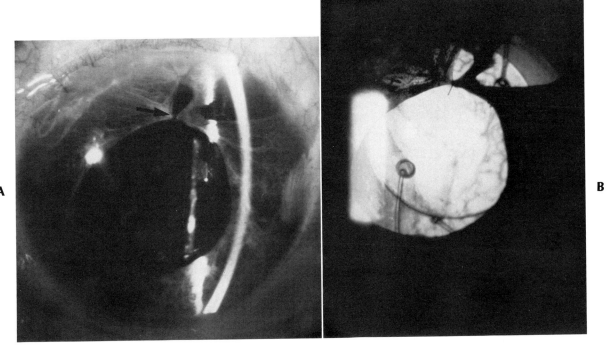

Fig. 7-35. A, Sutured iris *(arrow)* with a Shearing-type posterior chamber IOL in situ, in eye with previous excess mydriasis. **B,** Same eye, transilluminated. Note iris atrophy.

IRIS COLOBOMA

An eye with a previous sector iridectomy may be considered for the insertion of an iris-fixated lens implant, if the iris coloboma is repaired. In an ICCE, a 10-0 polypropylene suture is placed through the iris margins just above the sphincter. The suture is looped out of the eye, and the procedure is performed as described before. The ends of the suture can be left long to serve as a fixation suture. In an ECCE, the suture can be placed either before or after cataract extraction, as already noted (Fig. 7-36). A KPE is managed as previously described.

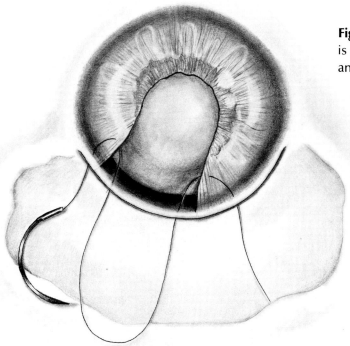

Fig. 7-36. A 10-0 polypropylene suture is placed through margins of coloboma and looped out of eye.

A surgical coloboma does not have to be repaired when a posterior or anterior chamber IOL is to be inserted, except for cosmetic reasons (Fig. 7-37). Some surgeons rotate a posterior chamber IOL so that its axis does not coincide with the surgical coloboma, to prevent the loops from dislocating anterior to the iris plane, a rare but undesirable situation (Fig. 7-38). An anterior chamber IOL must be inserted 90 degrees to the axis of the coloboma, lest a foot prolapse posteriorly, endangering the IOL fixation (see Fig. 8-5).

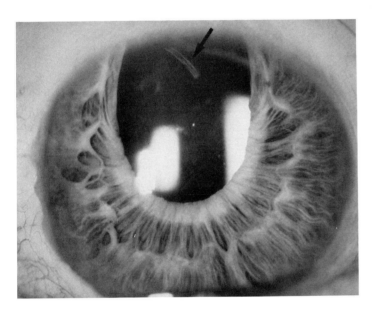

Fig. 7-37. Shearing-type IOL in situ in patient with sector iridectomy. Note superior loop *(arrow)*.

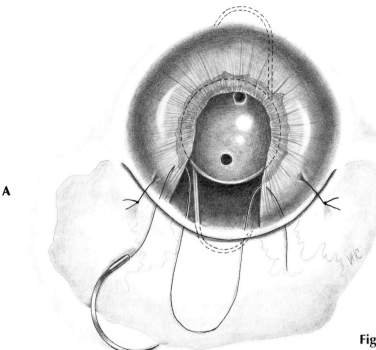

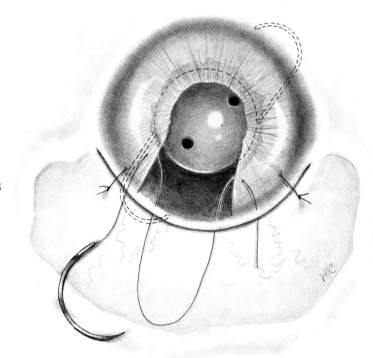

Fig. 7-38. A, Shearing-type posterior chamber IOL is inserted. **B,** Loops are rotated away from the coloboma. **C,** Coloboma is repaired.

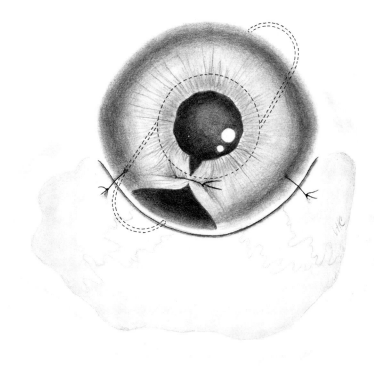

C

In eyes with a congenital coloboma, the surgeon should be ultraconservative. We believe the majority of these eyes are not candidates for IOL implantation. Many such eyes are amblyopic, and the patient's visual expectations may not be met. Also, the colobomas are generally inferior and slightly nasal; they would require an inferior section for closure or a McCannel suture technique (p. 248) followed by a conventional section (Fig. 7-39). If an ECCE or KPE is selected, the surgeon is cautioned that there may be a zonular defect corresponding to the general area of the coloboma. Its significance is that vitreous may appear while the anterior capsule and/or nucleus is being manipulated. If the ECCE or KPE is successfully performed, the posterior capsule may be suspect enough to contraindicate the implantation of a posterior chamber lens. Succinctly stated, the surgeon should be circumspect in operating on these cases, even if well versed in the procedure.

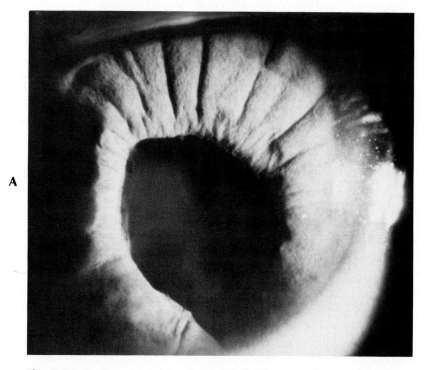

A

Fig. 7-39. A, Preoperative appearance of eye with congenital coloboma. **B,** Postoperative appearance of same eye following ICCE with superior section and radial iridotomy. **C,** Fundus view showing margins *(arrows)* of chorioretinal coloboma in same patient.

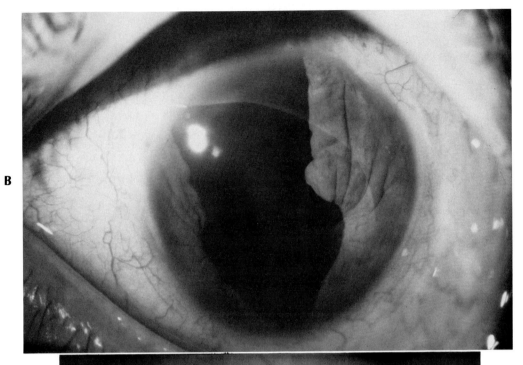

B

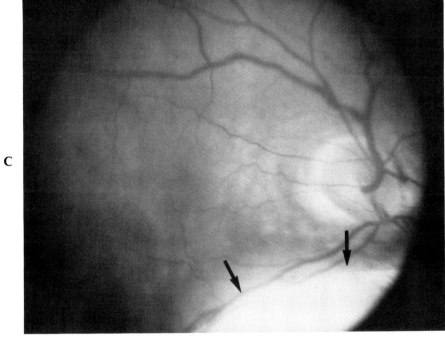

C

EYES WITH PREVIOUS PERIPHERAL IRIDECTOMIES

When an eye has had a previous peripheral iridectomy, the surgical technique is changed little, provided that the pupil dilates adequately, with or without the lysis of posterior synechiae. The initial KPE incision should not coincide with the peripheral iridectomy incision, since the desired 3.0-mm KPE incision, parallel to the iris, may not be feasible because of limbal distortion. Also, the ultrasonic probe may snag on the apex of the iridectomy, producing an iridodialysis. Similarly, the initial incision of an ECCE should be at a site different from that of the original iridectomy incision, to preclude complications during cystotome insertion and subsequent I/A procedures. In all types of cataract extraction, care should be exercised while enlarging the incision. If the intracorneal blade of the corneal-scleral section scissors inadvertently passes through the aperture of the peripheral iridectomy, and if the scissors are then closed with this blade posterior to the iris, a large iridodialysis will result, possibly with intraocular hemorrhage.

An iridodialysis will also occur if the apex of the peripheral iridectomy is snagged by the IOL while it is inserted. This can also happen when the peripheral iridectomy (Fig. 7-40) has resulted from closure of an iris coloboma (p. 212). This can be disastrous because the surgeon's view may be obscured by the advancing IOL covering the iridectomy. By the time the situation is discovered, there is a large iridodialysis, and the implant has to be withdrawn over the exposed anterior hyaloid face, in the case of an ICCE. A Sheets glide (p. 277) can also be used to bridge the iridectomy, but the best prevention is to remember this can happen and to exert the appropriate care.

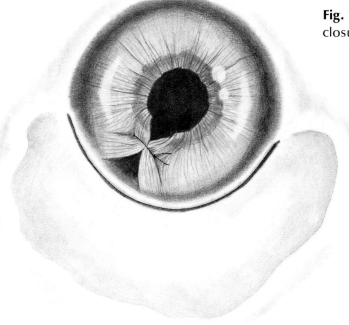

Fig. 7-40. Peripheral iridectomy formed after closure of surgical coloboma.

IRIS-FIXATION SUTURE PROBLEMS

The iris-fixation suture used with the Binkhorst iris clip and Worst Medallion IOLs can be entrapped by the loops of the IOL as it is inserted and becomes entwined around the IOL (Fig. 7-41). If this is recognized after the fixation suture has been tied, the situation should be left alone. When an entwined suture is noted before the fixation suture is tied, it should be remedied only if it can be done easily. If not, the fixation suture should be tied and the case proceeded with. Postoperatively, the surgeon's pride may be injured, but not the eye.

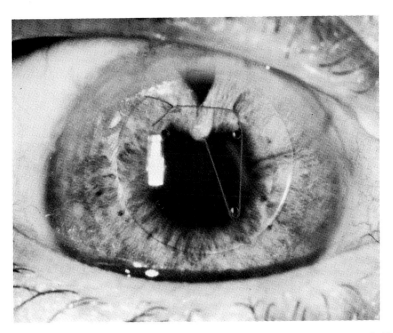

Fig. 7-41. Iris suture inadvertently tied around loop of implant. (From Jaffe, N.S., and others: Pseudophakos, St. Louis, 1978, The C.V. Mosby Co.)

The iris-fixation suture may be accidentally snatched by the surgeon or scrub nurse during the operation. The results run the gamut from minimal damage (Fig. 7-42) to avulsion of the iris (see Fig. 7-9), and the case will thereupon be managed according to the inflicted trauma. Attention to detail will prevent this complication. The surgeon and assistants should keep in mind the location of the iris suture, which should be moistened and adhered to the drapes. A loose end of a fixation suture swaying in the operating room's air flow is an invitation to this complication.

Iris-fixation sutures are not without risk, and the ophthalmologic profession's recognition of this has accelerated the trend to single-plane IOLs

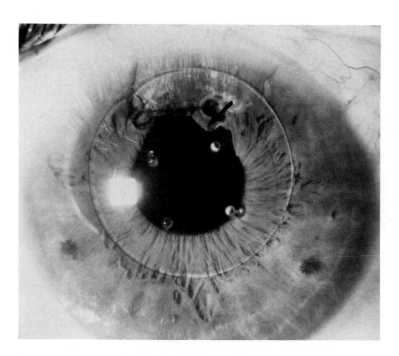

Fig. 7-42. Iris sphincter rupture *(arrow)* caused by accidental snatching on fixation suture.

that do not require iris suturing, i.e., posterior and anterior chamber lenses. However, an iris-fixation suture remains mandatory with a Worst Medallion IOL or a Binkhorst iris clip IOL inserted in conjunction with an ICCE.

Sometimes, long after the original surgery, an intracameral iris suture is noticed to have broken (Fig. 7-43). The breakage is actually degradation of the suture polymer, and thus far is reported only with nylon iris-fixation sutures (Fig. 7-44). We have seen this only with the Worst Medallion IOL, but there is no reason it could not occur with a Binkhorst iris clip or an iridoplasty suture. Two main considerations are how to manage the offending suture and whether the IOL should be refixated.

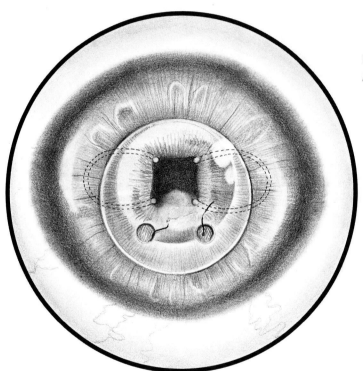

Fig. 7-43. Broken fixation suture in Worst Medallion IOL case.

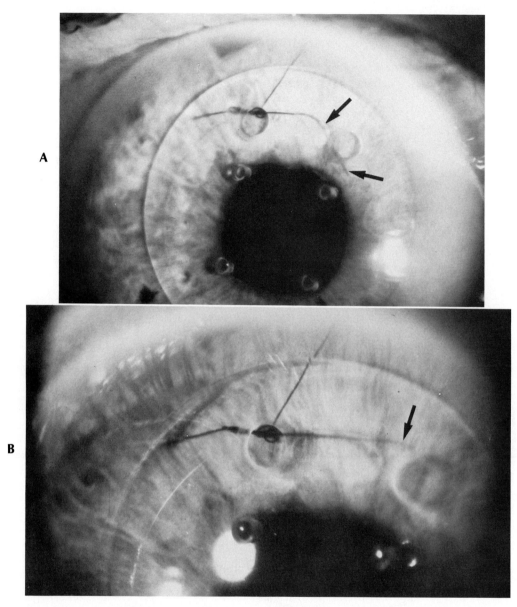

Fig. 7-44. A, Degradation of nylon iris-fixation suture. **B,** Same eye, higher magnification. Arrows indicate broken suture.

The broken suture should be removed only if it is excoriating the endothelium with resultant localized corneal edema, or if intermittent corneal touch is producing photophobia and ocular irritation (Fig. 7-45). The suture is removed by making a small incision at a convenient limbal site and removing the suture with Kelman-McPherson forceps under sodium hyaluronate or air, if required (Fig. 7-46). A noninvasive technique of shrinking the iris suture with an argon laser photocoagulation has also been reported.

When a degraded iris-fixation suture has been removed, should the IOL be refixated? The answer is *no* in the overwhelming majority of cases. If there are synechiae between the pupillary margin and the IOL, the lens will usually not dislocate. In cases without synechiae, the patient should be maintained with miotics. To minimize patient inconvenience, we recommend echothiophate iodide 0.03% every other night before retiring. For the infrequent case in which dislocation occurs, the lens is repositioned (Chapter 8) and a McCannel suture placed (p. 248).

A securely placed iris-fixation suture, nylon or polypropylene, could have been cut to leave an excessively long end. This can also excoriate the corneal endothelium. Since the suture is securely tied, the end cannot simply be withdrawn from the eye with forceps. If it is cut, how will the surgeon grasp the loose end and remove it from the anterior chamber? Removal can be achieved with a two-portal technique under sodium hyaluronate. One hand holds the suture with Kelman-McPherson forceps, while the other hand cuts it with either a razor knife of Vannas scissors. The loose end is removed with the Kelman-McPherson forceps. Rather than embark on a difficult surgical maneuver, it would be worthwhile initially to attempt laser shrinkage of the suture. It is best to remember that this situation should not arise if meticulous attention is given to *all* facets of the operation.

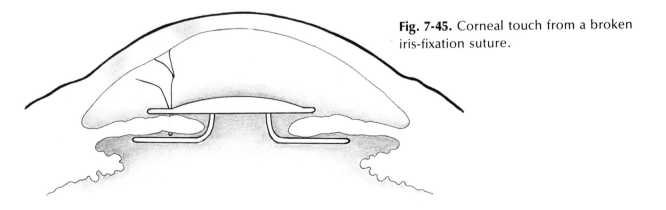

Fig. 7-45. Corneal touch from a broken iris-fixation suture.

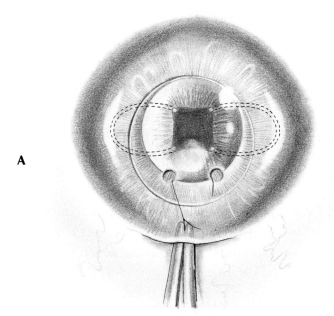

A

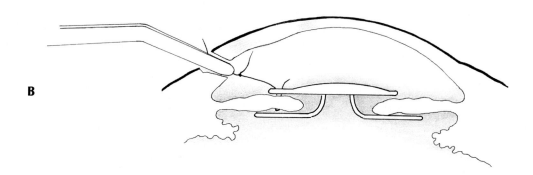

B

Fig. 7-46. A, Removal of broken fixation suture. **B,** Sagittal view of same procedure.

PUPILLARY BLOCK

We have arbitrarily included pupillary block in this chapter because its treatment may involve further iris surgery. Pupillary block occurs when there is inadequate communication between the posterior and anterior chambers, which impedes both aqueous circulation and the access of the aqueous to filtration at the angle. Aqueous accumulates in the posterior chamber, pushing forward the iris and shallowing the anterior chamber, with a concomitant rise in intraocular pressure. We have seen pupillary block glaucoma follow implantation of all types of IOLs and all types of cataract surgery, but we have the distinct impression that it occurs most frequently following an ICCE with Choyce-type anterior chamber IOLs (Fig. 7-47).

It is important, when making a diagnosis, to recognize that pupillary block exists with IOLs. Thereafter, attempts at pupillary dilatation may break the pupillary block so that no further treatment is required. Iris-fixated IOLs present a special problem, because mydriasis may precipitate dislocation. In these cases and in cases in which pupillary dilatation does not break the block, additional iris openings must be made. The argon laser may be used or surgical peripheral iridectomies performed.

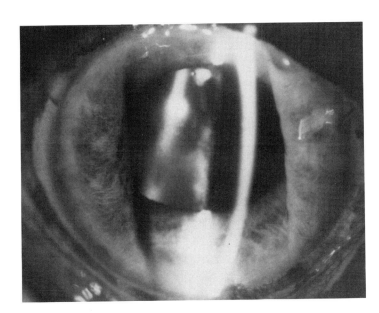

Fig. 7-47. Pupillary block with an anterior chamber IOL. (Courtesy Dr. Don Nicholson.)

We have previously alluded to the "instant" pupillary block sometimes seen with anterior chamber IOLs at insertion (Chapter 2) and the necessity for a midstromal iridotomy (see Fig. 2-15) to relieve internal iris prolapse. With postoperative pupillary block, especially with anterior chamber IOLs, the anterior chamber may not be uniformly shallow, but relatively formed in one area and virtually flat elsewhere. The laser or surgical iridotomy/iridectomy should be performed in the area of maximum anterior chamber shallowing, for it is in this area that the aqueous is trapped posterior to the iris by some quirk of aqueous dynamics.

Eight
Complications of lens implant position

The nature of malposition of a lens implant depends on the type of implant used and the method of securing it inside the eye. For example, one would see different clinical pictures with anterior chamber, iris-supported, iridocapsular, and posterior chamber lenses.

In general, malposition of a lens implant is caused by the following:

1. Too much air in the anterior chamber
2. Too wide a pupil as a result either of the rupture of a miotic pupil's sphincter during a cataract extraction or sphincter damage by a cryoprobe
3. Premature discontinuation of pilocarpine in the implants that are not secured by a fixation suture or device
4. Accidental use of mydriatics
5. Pupillary dilatation at night
6. Pupillary dilatation caused by excitement
7. Loop length of the implant being too short
8. Implant size being too small
9. Operative rupture of posterior capsule, or zonular dialysis
10. Ocular trauma

Dislocation of the whole IOL into the posterior chamber is treated as a separate topic in Chapter 10.

The anterior chamber lens implant is the least likely to malposition. The iris- and iridocapsular–supported lenses are the most likely to malposition. Posterior chamber lenses are intermediate in this respect.

ANTERIOR CHAMBER LENS IMPLANTS

An anterior chamber lens implant may spin like a propeller if it is too small. If too large, it can cause an iridodialysis or a detachment of the scleral spur. The implant may then migrate through this abnormal opening and decenter significantly. The location of the peripheral iridectomy is important. It must be placed at a safe distance away from the haptics of the implant. This is especially important with a three-point–fixation lens implant such as the Kelman lens. The trailing haptic is relatively narrow and can migrate through the iridectomy opening into the posterior chamber (Fig. 8-1) as noted in Chapter 2. The remainder of the implant might tilt and could result in corneal touch (Fig. 8-2) from IOL toe *A* (see Figs. 2-24 to 2-27).

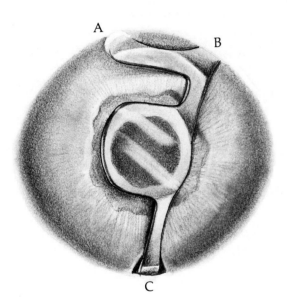

Fig. 8-1. Superior foot of Kelman IOL has migrated through peripheral iridectomy and destabilized the IOL.

Fig. 8-2. Destabilized IOL has rotated around its vertical axis causing toe *(A)* to touch corneal endothelium (sagittal view).

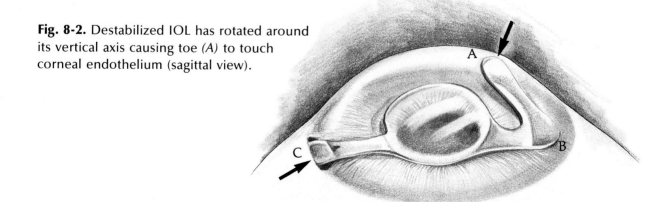

If one of the haptics of the anterior chamber lens has migrated through the peripheral iridectomy or through an inadvertent iridodialysis, it can be corrected by rotation of the implant to a safer position, if the IOL is correctly sized (Fig. 8-3). A corneoscleral incision must be made large enough so that the haptic can be exteriorized and the implant rotated. Once in the correct position, the scleral lip of the incision is retracted, and the proximal haptic is placed into the angle of the anterior chamber. Reposition by displacing the implant toward the distal part of the anterior chamber should not be attempted through a small incision. This could easily tear the iris root. The incision required for a Kelman lens is less than that for four-point–fixation anterior chamber lenses of the Choyce Mark VIII type. Sodium hyaluronate is useful in this situation.

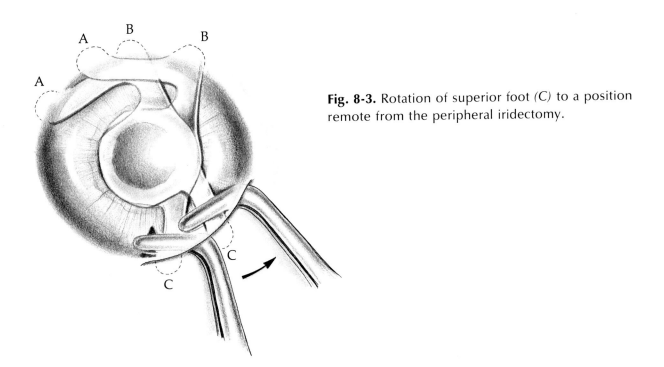

Fig. 8-3. Rotation of superior foot *(C)* to a position remote from the peripheral iridectomy.

When an anterior chamber IOL is too short, one of two things may happen. The IOL may change position several times in the postoperative period, eventually taking up a stable position and thereafter remaining immobile (Fig. 8-4). Or, the continued movement of the IOL may produce uveitis and/or place the IOL in a precarious position, necessitating IOL removal and possibly replacement. Fig. 8-5 shows a Kelman anterior chamber IOL, originally inserted temporally to bridge a preexistent sector iridectomy. The IOL has rotated placing foot *A* in the sector iridectomy. Surgical reintervention is indicated for this eye.

Iris tuck, discussed on p. 80, can be considered a complication of IOL position. If the patient exhibits symptoms of iris tuck from an excessively long anterior chamber IOL, it should be removed as described in Chapter 10. If intraoperative circumstances permit, we replace the offending IOL with another of the correct size.

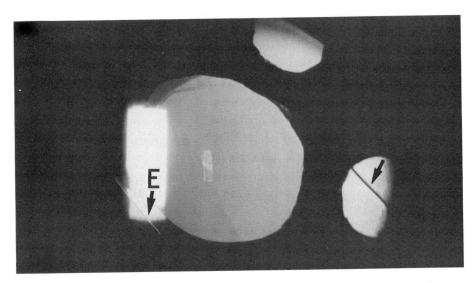

Fig. 8-4. A Choyce Mark VIII-type IOL inserted temporally. The IOL has "propellered" so that a foot is in the temporal iridectomy *(arrow)*, as seen in transillumination. The contralateral edge *(E)* can also be seen.

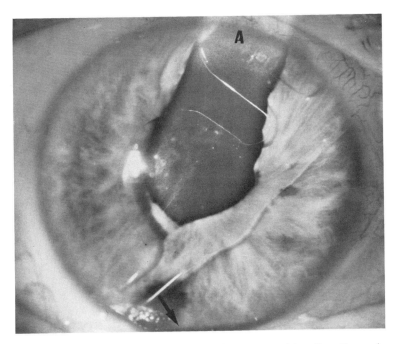

Fig. 8-5. Kelman anterior chamber IOL has rotated in direction of arrow. Foot *(A)* is in sector iridectomy.

IRIS AND IRIDOCAPSULAR LENS IMPLANTS

Most iris-supported lens implants should have some form of fixation to the iris, particularly with an ICCE. This is especially true for the Binkhorst 4-loop, Worst Medallion, Worst clip, and Fyodorov-Binkhorst lenses. The Copeland and Fyodorov Sputnik lenses are usually inserted safely without auxiliary iris fixation. Fixation to the iris does not ensure against malposition, but it virtually eliminates the possibility of dislocation into the vitreous.

If the superior haptic is fixated to the iris, the malposition usually involves the inferior haptic loops of the Binkhorst 4-loop and Worst Platina clip lenses. Both inferior loops may pass either in front of or behind the inferior iris in a Binkhorst 4-loop, the IOL may malposition, or the inferior foot may dislocate anterior to the iris, in the case of a Worst Platina. With the Worst Medallion lens, one or both horizontal loops may pass in front of the iris. There are more possibilities with the Fyodorov-Binkhorst and Copeland iris plane lenses, since the four haptics are located at 90-degree intervals from each other. The Fyodorov Sputnik lens, with its three loops and three struts, can present an even greater variety of malpositions.

The principles for reposition are the same for all these except the Copeland iris plane lens, which has no loops to work with.

Reposition is initially attempted pharmacologically. A short-acting mydriatic that is easily reversible, such as 10% phenylephrine or 1% tropicamide, is instilled. The patient's head is placed in a position determined by the portion of the implant that has subluxated. As soon as the pupil dilates enough that the distal portion of the subluxated haptic clears the iris margin, the patient's head is placed in an appropriate position (e.g., head back if both inferior loops of a Binkhorst 4-loop lens are in front of the iris, head forward if they are behind). A miotic solution, such as 2% pilocarpine or 0.12% to 0.25% echothiophate iodide, is placed in the eye (Fig. 8-6).

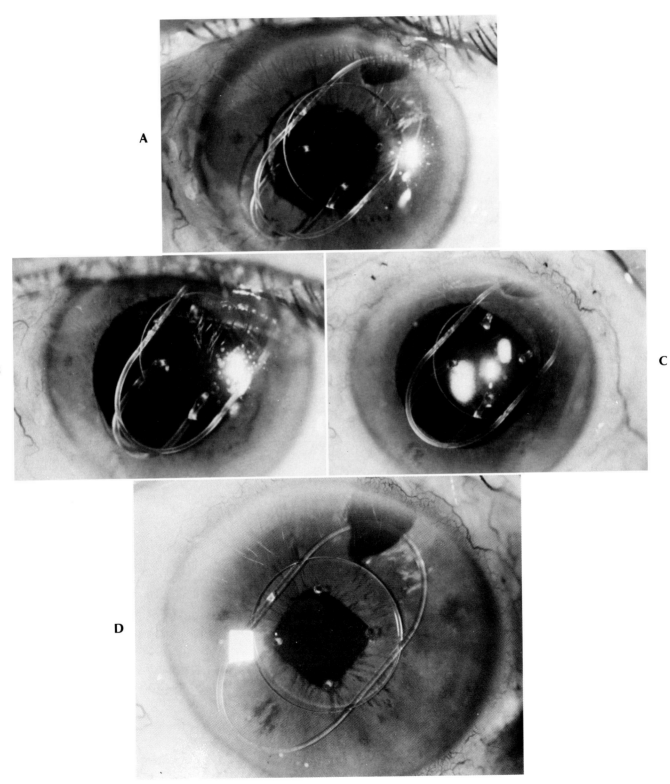

Fig. 8-6. A, Spontaneous dislocation of Binkhorst iris clip IOL. Both inferior loops anterior to iris. **B,** Pupil dilated with 10% phenylephrine solution. **C,** Posterior inferior loop posterior to iris. **D,** IOL in situ after miosis with 0.12% echothiophate iodide solution. (From Jaffe, N.S.: Cataract surgery and its complications, ed. 3, St. Louis, 1981, The C.V. Mosby Co.)

If pharmacology fails, instrumental repositioning must be used. This may be done as an office or outpatient hospital procedure. A spatula or a disposable 27-gauge needle attached to a syringe is used. A cotton stick applicator soaked in 10% cocaine solution is applied to the limbus at a location optimum for entry into the anterior chamber. A retrobulbar injection of an anesthetic mixture is usually not required. If the inferior loops of a Binkhorst 4-loop lens are behind the iris, the 27-gauge needle enters just inside the limbus from a temporal position, with 0.12-mm fixation forceps fixating the globe. The needle passes across the anterior chamber until it is positioned so that the optic can be displaced toward the 12 o'clock position. As soon as the distal end of the anterior inferior loop clears the pupillary border, the needle is withdrawn to the point of entry, but not removed from the eye. This permits the implant to move toward the 6 o'clock position with the inferior portion of the iris safely positioned between the two inferior haptic loops. When both inferior feet of the Binkhorst IOL are anterior to the iris and fail to reposition pharmacologically (Fig. 8-7), a similar surgical maneuver is used for repositioning. Fig 8-8 shows the dislocated superior feet. A spatula or needle is passed into the anterior chamber between the loops of the IOL, and maneuvers the IOL into position with the surgeon using the optic insertion of the posterior inferior loop as the fulcrum (Fig. 8-9).

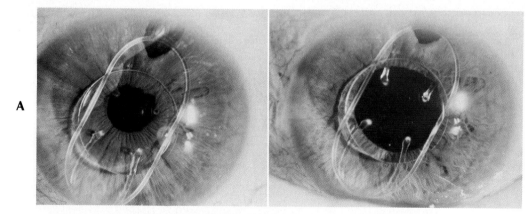

Fig. 8-7. A, Dislocation of Binkhorst iris clip IOL. **B,** Maximal mydriasis insufficient for pharmacologic repositioning of inferior loops. Surgical intervention required. (From Jaffe, N.S., and others: Pseudophakos, St. Louis, 1978, The C.V. Mosby Co.)

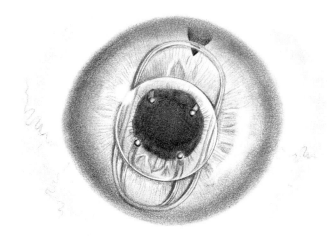

Fig. 8-8. Anterior dislocation of inferior feet of Binkhorst iris clip IOL.

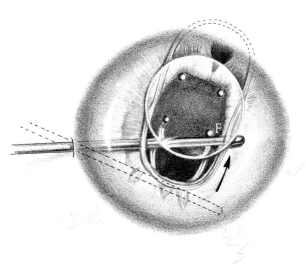

Fig. 8-9. Spatula inserted through a stab wound in limbus. IOL maneuvered into position using optic insertion of posterior inferior loop as fulcrum *(F)*.

The same principle applies to the repositioning of one of the horizontal loops of a Worst Medallion lens (Fig. 8-10). In this case, the needle or spatula enters vertically, rather than horizontally, either from above or below. The instrument passes across the anterior chamber until it can displace the optic so that the distal margin of the subluxated haptic clears the pupillary border (Fig. 8-11), whereupon the loop is pushed posteriorly by the instrument, so that the dislocated loop can pass behind the iris.

If an iris-fixation suture was not used primarily, a McCannel suture may be used at this time to secure the anterior superior loop of the Binkhorst 4-loop lens. If repeated subluxations of the inferior loops have occurred, a McCannel suture may be used to secure the anterior inferior loop of the im-

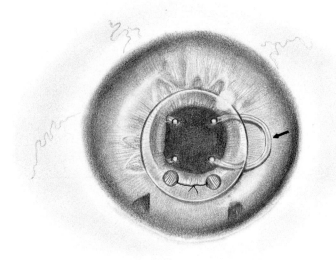

Fig. 8-10. Dislocated loop of Worst Medallion IOL *(arrow).*

Fig. 8-11. Dislocated loop of IOL maneuvered until its apex clears pupillary margin. The loop is allowed to spring into position posterior to the iris, aided by posterior pressure from the spatula. Arrow shows motion.

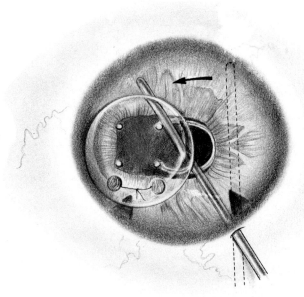

plant. The McCannel technique and its variations (discussed later in this chapter) are useful in all chronically dislocating looped IOLs.

Reposition of a Copeland iris plane lens cannot be performed with a needle as it can with other iris-supported lenses, since the haptics are solid (Fig. 8-12). If pharmacologic repositioning fails, as usually occurs with this type of IOL, the patient should be taken to the operating room. An adequate stab wound is made at the limbus just over the 12 o'clock haptic, if this haptic is anterior to the iris. Otherwise, another site is chosen where a haptic is anterior to the iris. The incision should be large enough to permit entry of a Clayman or Shepard forceps. The haptic is grasped with these forceps so that the implant can be properly repositioned (Fig. 8-13).

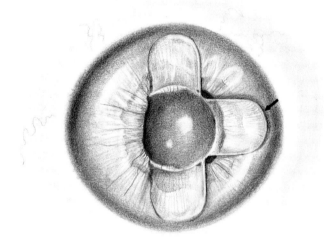

Fig. 8-12. Dislocated foot of Copeland IOL *(arrow).*

Fig. 8-13. Copeland IOL maneuvered into correct position with Clayman forceps. Arrow shows motion.

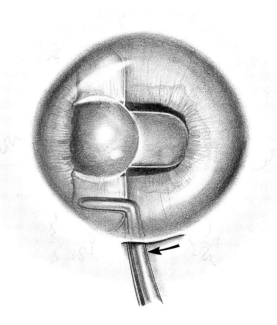

Dislocations occur for which the surgeon must devise a technique. Fig. 8-14 shows a Fyodorov Sputnik IOL completely dislocated into the anterior chamber. Since this IOL has three posterior loops and three anterior pintles (p. 119), a two-instrument technique is used for repositioning.

When decentration occurs without dislocation, it nearly always does so within the first 6 postoperative months. It may be caused by iris incarceration, iris prolapse, peripheral anterior synechiae, an atonic pupil, too tight a suture used for fixation to the iris, or vitreous strands in the anterior chamber. After an ECCE, decentration may result from an asymmetric adhesion

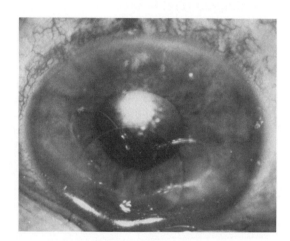

Fig. 8-14. Fyodorov Sputnik IOL, completely dislocated into the anterior chamber.

Fig. 8-15. Sagittal view of vitreous incarcerated in cataract section, decentering optic against corneal endothelium.

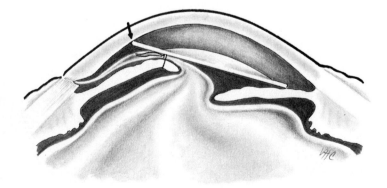

of the loop supports to residual capsulolenticular material. The most frequent case of decentration is fibroplasia of vitreous left in the anterior chamber when operative loss of vitreous has occurred. If there is extensive incarceration of vitreous in the wound, the implant may become so decentered that the optical portion or an anterior loop (as in a Binkhorst 4-loop lens) touches the cornea or comes dangerously close to it (Fig. 8-15). This must be surgically corrected by removing the offending vitreous (Fig. 8-16) and repositioning the implant (Fig. 8-17).

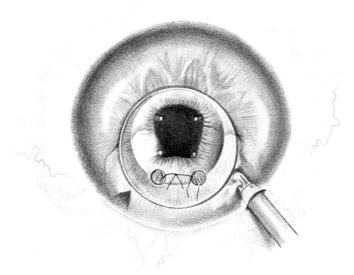

Fig. 8-16. Incarcerated vitreous removed with vitreophage.

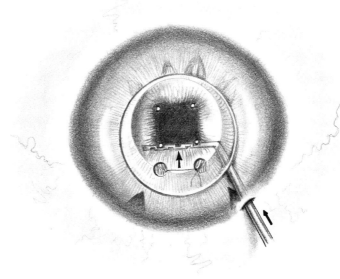

Fig. 8-17. Optic repositioned away from the cornea by a notched spatula. Arrow shows motion.

The possibility of malposition or dislocation of an iridocapsular lens implant is less than with an iris-supported lens because of the greater reliability of capsular fixation. However, if capsule rupture with or without vitreous loss should occur, it would be dangerous to use an iridocapsular implant, since an iris-fixation suture or clip is generally not used. Repositioning is performed exactly as described for iris-supported lenses with one exception. If an iridocapsular lens is recovered from the vitreous, it should be removed from the eye. If the optic passes behind the eye so that the entire implant is in the posterior chamber with an intact posterior capsule, it may be left in this position (Fig. 8-18).

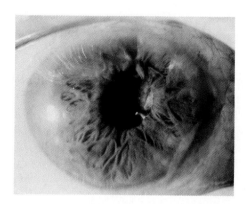

Fig. 8-18. Optic of Binkhorst iridocapsular IOL dislocated into posterior chamber following an ECCE with an iridoplasty. (From Jaffe, N.S., and others: Pseudophakos, St. Louis, 1978, The C.V. Mosby Co.)

POSTERIOR CHAMBER LENS IMPLANTS

The four kinds of malpositions of posterior chamber lens implants are these:

1. Decentration
2. Pupil capture
3. Windshield wiper syndrome
4. Sunset syndrome

Decentration may result in the edge of the optic reaching the area of the pupil. It rarely causes a serious disturbance in vision. If it remains fixed in this position and is kept under observation, it requires no treatment. This condition can be seen during surgery and remedied by manipulating the IOL with either a Jaffe hook or a Clayman guide placed in the optic bore holes. If, on recentering the optic, it immediately decenters when the instrument is disengaged, one loop is probably in the capsular bag and the other in the ciliary sulcus. We recommend no treatment. Apparent decentration may be seen from *reverse iris tuck* (p. 80). With posterior chamber IOLs, especially those with anterior angulated loops (p. 148), the posterior peripheral aspect of the iris may be tucked between the apex of the loop and the ciliary sulcus. This peaks the pupil in the axis of the loops and gives the impression of decentration. Reverse iris tuck is easily overcome by rotating the optic clockwise, which releases the tucked iris and permits the pupil to resume its normal shape.

Pupil capture is caused by a portion or all of the optic of the lens passing anteriorly to the iris (Fig. 8-19). It occurs less frequently with the Kratz modification of the loops of a Shearing-type lens. It must be corrected early, or else adhesion of the iris to the posterior capsule prevents repositioning of the optic. The pupil is dilated with 1% tropicamide while the patient is supine. The optic usually falls back into the posterior chamber. The pupil is then constricted by 2% pilocarpine or 0.12% to 0.25% echothiophate iodide. If capture recurs as the pupil constricts (Fig. 8-20), a spatula or a 27-gauge disposable needle on a syringe is used to tap the optic into position through a corneal stab wound just inside the limbus (Fig. 8-21). If capture is seen after adhesions have formed, and the pupil cannot be dilated in the area of the capture, repositioning should not be attempted. Except for the esthetic disadvantage, pupillary capture is not a serious problem.

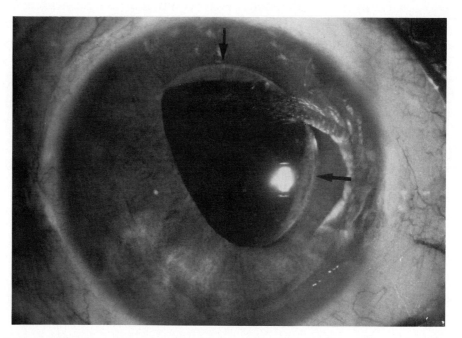

Fig. 8-19. Pupillary capture with a Shearing posterior chamber IOL. Note edge of optic *(arrows)* anterior to iris.

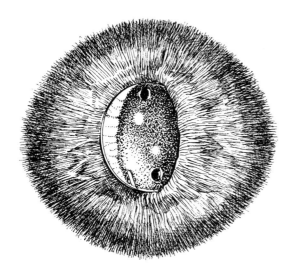

Fig. 8-20. Recapture of optic by constricting pupil.

Fig. 8-21. Optic tapped into position with a spatula. Optic should be held in posterior chamber until iris is constricted over it by means of intracameral acetylcholine.

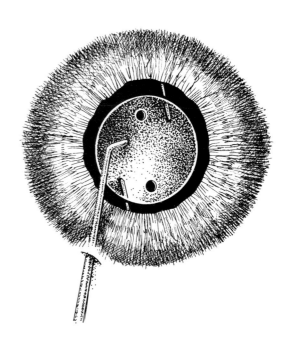

Windshield wiper syndrome usually results from an implant that is too small for the eye. The superior loop does not fixate well in the superior cilary sulcus. Therefore the upper portion of the implant has a pendular movement with ocular rotation (Fig. 8-22). If disturbing, it can be corrected with a McCannel suture. We have seen this syndrome occur after a secondary implantation of a posterior chamber IOL has been performed. Presumably there is no adhesion of the IOL to the posterior capsule. In primary posterior chamber IOL implantation, over 95% of the IOLs adhere to the posterior capsule in addition to being fixated at the ciliary sulcus.

The sunset syndrome is the most serious malposition problem of a posterior chamber lens. It may occur early or late in the postoperative period. When discovered early, it usually has resulted from a zonular dialysis unrecognized at the time of surgery, or has been assumed to be a mild decentration problem. When discovered late (months to years after the initial surgery), it may have been caused by trauma or by rubbing the eye, which can cause a zonular dialysis. This is less likely to occur if the loops of a Shearing lens are rotated to the horizontal position, or if lenses with more flexible loops are used (e.g., Sinskey, Simcoe, Clayman).

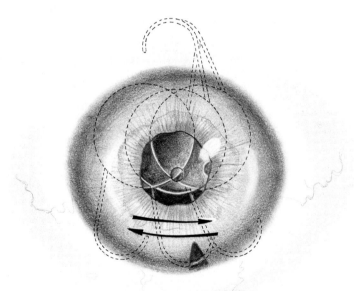

Fig. 8-22. Concept of windshield wiper syndrome. Lens pivots to and fro with ocular movement.

When the optic begins to sink toward the 6 o'clock position, it should be observed carefully. It may finally come to rest without sinking further. In many cases, it will continue its descent until most of the lens is in the vitreous.

The sunset syndrome may be corrected in any of three ways. A Jaffe hook or Clayman guide is inserted into one of the drill holes near the edge of the optic. The optic is pulled toward the 12 o'clock position (Fig. 8-23). When it is well centered, a McCannel suture is used to ensure fixation. An alternate method is to create a complete pupil capture by maneuvering the optic anterior to the iris with a Jaffe or Sinskey hook. It results in a cat's-eye (vertical ellipse) pupil, but the lens can remain safely in this position (Fig. 8-24). If the lens drops considerably into the vitreous, and vitreous fills the pupillary space and perhaps the anterior chamber, the lens should be removed. Following a partial anterior vitrectomy, an anterior chamber or iris-supported lens may be used at the surgeon's discretion.

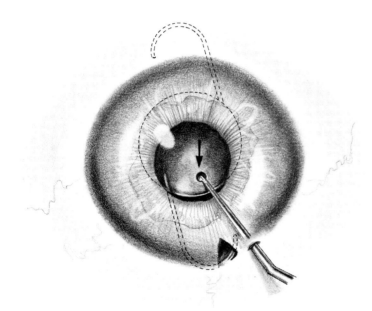

Fig. 8-23. Inferiorly displaced posterior chamber IOL being drawn superiorly so that optic is in pupil and apex of superior loop is at peripheral iridectomy and accessible for a McCannel suture as required.

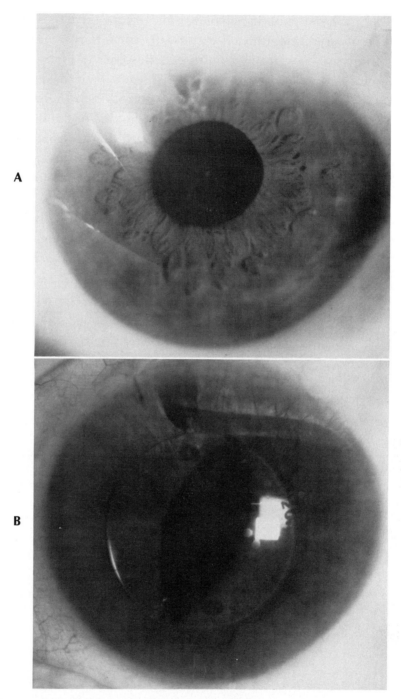

Fig. 8-24. A, A dislocated posterior chamber IOL. The optic is no longer in the pupil, leaving the visual axis aphakic. **B,** Same eye. The optic has been drawn into the pupil, and an iatrogenic pupillary capture has been created, giving a vertically oval pupil.

Malpositions of a posterior chamber lens are less frequent when capsular bag fixation is used, but the surgery is more complex, and the possibility of zonular dialysis still exists.

The insertion of a posterior chamber IOL requires an intact posterior capsule. If, at the conclusion of an ECCE or KPE, there is capsular rupture or dehiscence of the posterior capsule, the insertion of the posterior chamber IOL may have to be abandoned in favor of either an iris-fixated or an anterior chamber IOL, the latter being our preference. This is to prevent a sunset syndrome.

Rarely, a dialysis of the posterior capsule is noted *after* the posterior chamber IOL has been inserted. This places the surgeon in a predicament because, if no action is taken, the IOL could dislocate into the posterior chamber (p. 275). Alternatively, removal of the IOL may be accompanied by vitreous loss. We elect not to remove the IOL, but we take the precaution of suturing it to the iris. If either loop can be safely rotated to the peripheral iridectomy, it should be done (Fig. 8-23). The loop is externalized about 2 mm, so that its apex overlies the ciliary sulcus. A 10-0 polypropylene suture (e.g., Ethicon D-2794) is passed around the loop, posterior to anterior, and through the iris at the left lateral margin of the iridectomy. The suture is *tightly* tied and trimmed. The superior loop is reposited into the posterior chamber through the aperture of the peripheral iridectomy, with care taken that the suture does not slide superiorly up the loop. If that occurs, the optic will position inferiorly and fail to fill the pupil.

McCANNEL METHOD

The McCannel suture technique has been mentioned many times in this text; it is an ingenious method for placing an intracameral fixation suture with a closed chamber technique. A stab wound is made just within the limbus adjacent to clear cornea closest to the position where the suture will end up being tied to the iris (Fig. 8-25). A double-arm 9-0 or 10-0 polypropylene suture on a half-curve cutting edge needle is passed through this incision, through the iris (Fig. 8-26), around the loop, which may be anterior or posterior to the iris (according to the implant type), back out through the

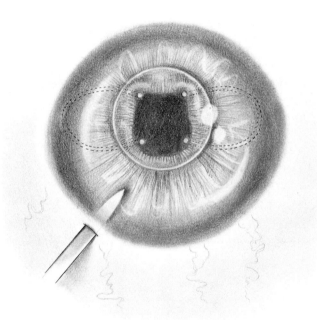

Fig. 8-25. Stab wound in surgical limbus.

Fig. 8-26. Needle is passed through incision and through iris.

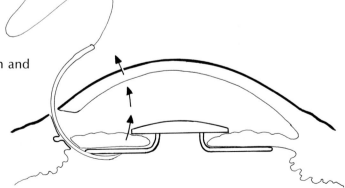

iris, and finally out through the cornea at any point where the needle ends up (Fig. 8-27). At this point we have a suture that is passing through the stab wound, through the iris, around a loop, through the iris again, and out through the cornea. The needle is cut off from the leading end of the suture that has emerged from the cornea. Left outside the cornea after the needle is cut off are 5.0 to 7.5 cm of suture. A small iris hook is introduced through the stab wound, and the free end of the suture is grasped and withdrawn from the eye through the stab wound (Fig. 8-28). Both ends of the suture

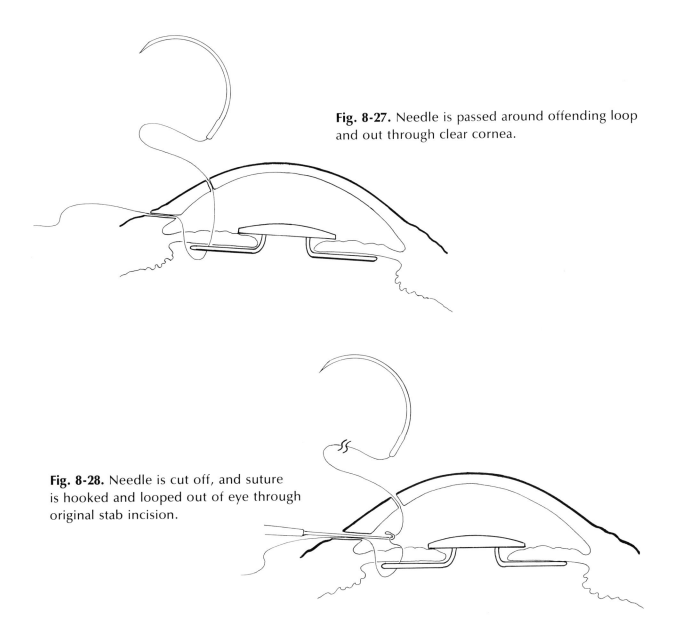

Fig. 8-27. Needle is passed around offending loop and out through clear cornea.

Fig. 8-28. Needle is cut off, and suture is hooked and looped out of eye through original stab incision.

emerge from the stab wound; these two ends are tied together with four knots. This brings the loop and iris up to the stab wound (Fig. 8-29). The suture knot must be free from any tissue fragments at the stab wound site. The suture is cut close to the knot. The iris and the sutured loop will then retract into the anterior chamber (Fig. 8-30).

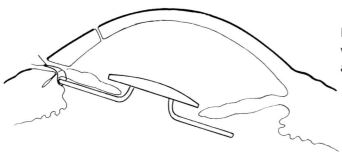

Fig. 8-29. Suture is tied and trimmed at stab wound. Care is taken to avoid incarcerating any tissue in the knot.

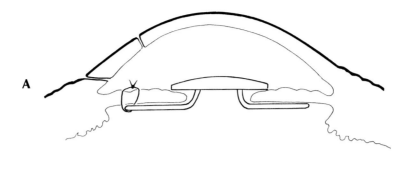

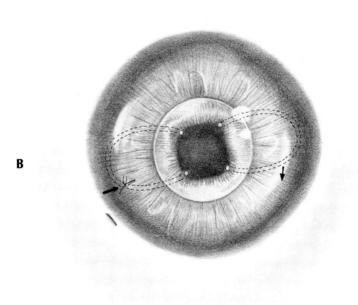

Fig. 8-30. A, Appearance of McCannel suture in situ (sagittal views).
B, McCannel suture *(left arrow).* Note proximity to stab incision. Arrow on right shows superior direction of repositioned IOL.

Nine
Complications of media

In this chapter, complications as they pertain to an IOL in situ are considered, starting with the anterior segment and progressing posteriorly. Corneal complications have been discussed in Chapter 6.

HYPHEMA

Hyphema can be a serious intraoperative complication of IOL surgery because it can impede the surgeon's view of IOL insertion and placement. Blood clots adherent to the iris inhibit pupillary constriction, which is especially necessary to the fixation and centration of iris-supported IOLs. The most common source of intraoperative hyphema is bleeding from the incision, especially in the presence of an excessively posterior section. The 3 o'clock and 9 o'clock aspects of the incision are particularly susceptible because of their perfusion from the long choroidal artery and its anterior tributaries (see Fig. 1-10). A wet-field coagulator is an excellent achiever of hemostasis, which should be obtained both before and after making the incision (see Fig. 1-15).

Intraoperative hyphema can also be secondary to an iridodialysis (p. 190) or an excessively basal iridectomy. The best treatment is prevention; however, the wet-field coagulator can be used intracamerally if the source of bleeding can be identified. If it cannot, try hemostasis with gentle irrigation. If the bleeding is not contained, the eye should be temporarily closed and repressurized. Another source of intraoperative hyphema is anticoagulant therapy, so specific inquiries should be made concerning the patient's medication history.

Postoperative hyphema occurs after IOL surgery for all the reasons it occurs after routine cataract surgery. There is an additional situation peculiar to IOLs, known as the uveitis-glaucoma-hyphema (UGH) syndrome, caused by imperfectly manufactured IOLs. The UGH syndrome usually requires IOL removal; this topic is discussed in Chapter 10. There is no concensus about the management of postoperative hyphema, and the treatment regimens range from complete bed rest to unlimited activity. Some surgeons advocate mydriasis, others miosis, and yet another school no topical treatment; but most would concur on the desirability of controlling intraocular pressure (Fig. 9-1).

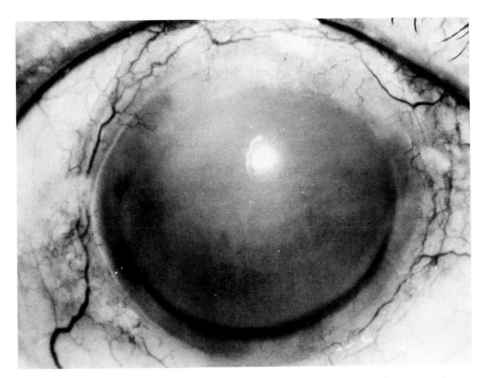

Fig. 9-1. Bloodstaining of the cornea after hyphema and elevated intraocular pressure following cataract surgery. (From Jaffe, N.S.: Cataract surgery and its complications, ed. 3, St. Louis, 1981, The C.V. Mosby Co.)

A postoperative hyphema occupying up to 75% of the anterior chamber will clear spontaneously if there has been no new bleeding. In our experience, this will occur with or without limitation of activity or topical treatment, but the hyphema will persist longer when an IOL is in situ. It is interesting to observe that the last remnants of the blood clot will often adhere to the IOL optic rather than in the inferior angle. The surgeon should be cautious in the use of mydriasis in postoperative hyphema when an IOL is in situ. The pupil does not dilate well when hyphema is present, but any dilatation that is produced could subluxate an iris-fixated IOL.

Presented with a hyphema greater than 75% of the anterior chamber, the surgeon must decide whether to intervene surgically. The problem with large hyphemas is that they obstruct the trabeculum, through which the degraded blood is cleared by the aqueous flow; hence the degraded blood tends to persist. For the same reason intraocular pressure is usually elevated, and the surgeon must consider the risks of corneal bloodstaining and the possibility of damage to the posterior segment, such as vein occlusion or ischemic optic neuropathy. Certainly, it is prudent initially to treat these large hyphemas with observation and the appropriate ocular antihypertensive agents, but if excessive intraocular pressures persist and there is no tendency of the blood to reabsorb, then surgical intervention is indicated. It is difficult to be dogmatic about the postoperative day on which surgical intervention becomes mandatory, but we feel the range is three to seven days depending on the clinical picture. A total hyphema ("eight ball hemorrhage") would be earlier in the range and a 75% hyphema would be later.

There are various methods to surgically manage hyphemas, and before discussing two of these let us remind the reader of the obvious: the blood in the anterior chamber is clotted and tenaciously adherent to the iris and IOL; therefore patience and caution should be exercised during the procedure. Every effort should be made to lower the intraocular pressure before starting the procedure. To decompress *suddenly* a recently operated on and hence inflamed eye with excessive intraocular pressure is an invitation for an expulsive hemorrhage. If the pressure cannot be lowered preoperatively, then with the initial incision the globe should be *slowly* decompressed.

Two surgical methods for management of hyphema are wash-out and irrigation/aspiration. In the former, two 22-gauge disposable needles are obtained. One is connected to a 500-cc bottle of balanced saline solution or its equivalent. This needle is inserted through the surgical limbus into the anterior chamber at the 9 o'clock position, making no conjunctival flap and steadied with the surgeon's right hand. The second needle, unattached to any instrument or tubing, is passed with the left hand into the anterior chamber at the 3 o'clock position, also with no conjunctival flap. The irrigation bottle is opened, and irrigating solution is permitted to flow into the anterior chamber through the right-hand needle and out of the anterior chamber through the left-hand needle. The fluid flow within the anterior chamber washes out the hyphema through the left-hand needle. The emanating fluid is xanthochromic and occasionally blood tinged. Either of the needles can be used to agitate the hyphema to expedite its wash-out. The advantages of a wash-out procedure are that no special equipment or conjunctival flap is required, and that suture closure of the two stab incisions is generally unnecessary. Also, the initial cataract incision is avoided. The disadvantage is that the procedure is slow, and large amounts of irrigating fluid may have to be run through the anterior chamber.

Irrigation and aspiration of a hyphema is relatively rapid and can be performed with the CooperVision Systems/Cavitron equipment (p. 17). A superior rectus suture is placed (p. 3), and the conjunctival flap is retracted to expose the original incision. A 3-mm section is required through which the I/A handpiece is inserted (p. 31), and the appropriate sutures are removed from the initial incision. If hyphema completely obscures all details of the anterior chamber, gently irrigate the anterior chamber at the incision so that some idea can be obtained of the chamber depth because the insertion of the I/A tip could cause further damage. Enter the eye with the handpiece in position 1 (irrigation only). Once in the eye, go into position 2 (irrigation and aspiration) and evacuate the hyphema. Adherent fibrin and blood clots may have to be mechanically stripped from intracameral structures by engagement at the aspiration orifice and mechanical debridement, at which point they will be easily aspirated. The I/A handpiece is withdrawn and the incision is sutured. Some hyphemas can be extremely difficult to break up, and if irrigation/aspiration is not proceeding well, a vitreophage should be used. A vitreous hemorrhage might accompany a hyphema; this is discussed later in this chapter.

LENS PRECIPITATES

Pigment and inflammatory precipitates are sometimes seen on the surfaces of an IOL, especially during the immediate postoperative period. These usually clear spontaneously and are rarely a cause of vision loss. Persistent lens precipitates, assuming an IOL of good quality and an absence of other ocular disease, usually clear with topical steroid therapy. However, when the lens precipitates are part of a chronic inflammatory ocular syndrome (p. 273) induced by a faulty IOL, they do not clear, and IOL removal may be indicated (Fig. 9-2). There usually is decreased vision in these patients, but it is difficult to decide whether the lens precipitates, concomitant CME, or both are culpable.

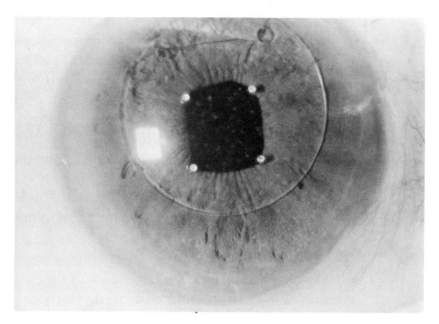

Fig. 9-2. Pigment deposits on a metal-looped Medallion-style IOL. (From Jaffe, N.S., and others: Pseudophakos, St. Louis, 1978, The C.V. Mosby Co.)

OPACIFICATION OF POSTERIOR CAPSULE

Posterior capsular opacification is not a media opacity peculiar to IOL surgery but rather is associated with ECCE. It has been estimated that more than 30% of posterior capsules will ultimately opacify and, given the growing trend to extracapsular surgery, these opacifications will become an ever-increasing cause of surgical reintervention. Not all capsular opacifications are in the visual axis, and those that are may affect the vision only minimally. The surgeon will have to decide when to intervene, taking into account the patient's visual needs. These opacities give symptoms similar to those of posterior subcapsular cataracts, and the patient's vision, in a dimly lit examining room, may be deceptively good (Fig. 9-3).

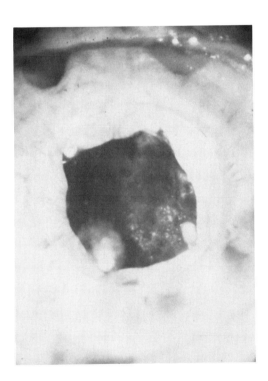

Fig. 9-3. Opacification of posterior capsule following an ECCE in patient with a Binkhorst iridocapsular IOL.

When a discission is indicated, the presence of an IOL in situ modifies the procedure slightly. We fashion a hook on a 25- or 27-gauge needle as described in Chapter 1 (p. 23). This needle is attached to intravenous tubing which is attached to a bottle of balanced saline or lactated Ringer's solution. Better maneuverability of the needle is obtained if it is attached to the Cooper-Vision Systems/Cavitron irrigation handpiece (p. 23), if that is available. For a right eye, we enter the anterior chamber at the 9 o'clock position with a razor knife at the limbus, just anterior to the conjunctival insertion. The knife enters more easily if counterpressure is applied at the 3 o'clock position by grasping conjunctiva and Tenon's capsule with 0.12-mm forceps. When discissing a left eye, we enter the anterior chamber at the 3 o'clock position and apply the counterpressure at the 9 o'clock position.

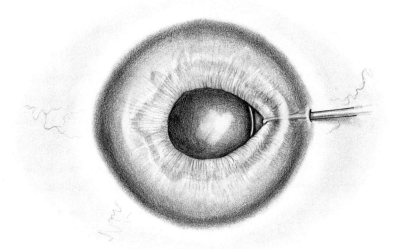

Fig. 9-4. Iris is retracted with hooked discission needle to expose lateral edge of posterior chamber IOL.

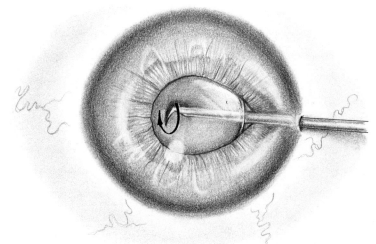

Fig. 9-5. Needle is slid behind IOL and turned posteriorly to engage capsule.

Anterior chamber, iris-fixated, and iridocapsular IOLs occupy positions within the anterior chamber that permit easy access to the posterior capsule. A posterior chamber IOL presents a different situation. Here, the iris must be retracted to expose the edge of the IOL, under which the 27-gauge discission needle is insinuated. Specifically, the needle is passed into the anterior chamber with the hook horizontal. The hook is then turned so the point is posterior and used to retract the iris until the lateral edge of the IOL is seen (Fig. 9-4). The needle is again turned horizontally and passed between the back surface of the optic and the posterior capsule, across the pupillary aperture to the contralateral pupillary margin at least 2 mm lateral to the center of the pupil. The needle is then turned posteriorly (Fig. 9-5), and the posterior capsule is engaged and discissed by drawing the needle back toward the incision site (Fig. 9-6). The discission should be made at least 4 mm long. On completion of the discission, the needle is turned hori-

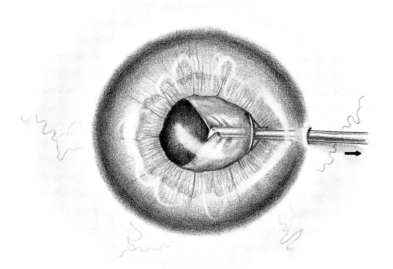

Fig. 9-6. Capsule is discissed by drawing discission needle toward stab incision.

zontally and withdrawn from the anterior chamber (Fig. 9-7). A suture is rarely required. The maneuver is identical for anterior chamber, iris-fixated, and iridocapsular IOLs, except that there is no need for iris retraction (Fig. 9-8).

A primary posterior capsulectomy (discission) is discussed in Chapter 1 (p. 35), but a few additional points need clarification. If the posterior capsule is engaged exactly in the optical center and discissed, a V-shaped paracentral discission will result, which still may partially obstruct the visual axis (Fig. 9-9). The reason is that the posterior capsule "gives" in the direction the needle is being withdrawn, as it is initially discissed. It is for this reason we advocate discissing from 2 mm peripheral to the optical center to 2 mm beyond, on the other side of the optical center. This applies to both primary and secondary discissions.

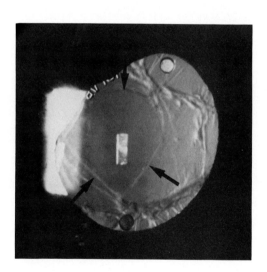

Fig. 9-7. Discission *(arrows)* as a second procedure in an eye with a posterior chamber IOL. Shown in transillumination.

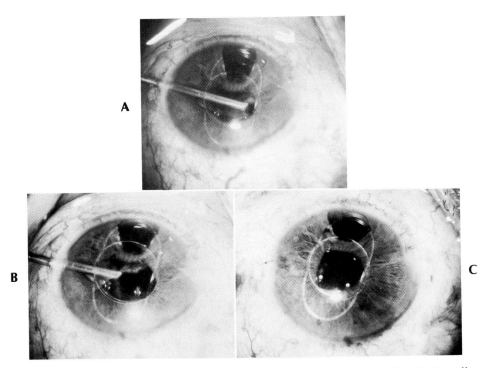

Fig. 9-8. A, Capsule is engaged posterior to Binkhorst iris clip IOL. **B,** Needle is drawn toward stab incision. **C,** Appearance after discission. (From Jaffe, N.S., and others: Pseudophakos, St. Louis, 1978, The C.V. Mosby Co.)

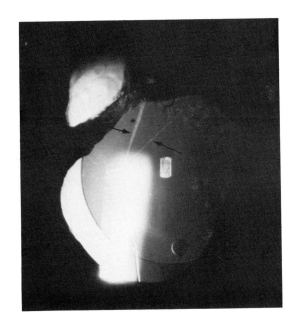

Fig. 9-9. Paracentral discission *(arrows)* behind posterior chamber IOL in eye with iris atrophy.

Another point to consider in secondary discissions is whether access to the posterior capsule is impeded by posterior synechiae. When this occurs, it is most frequently seen between the superior iris and posterior capsule, since this is the area of greater surgical manipulation and also the area of capsular cul-de-sac, wherein surgical accessibility is more limited and hence more likely to harbor residual cortex. If an attempt is made to perform a secondary discission through the original peripheral iridectomy, the advancing discission needle could be obstructed by synechiae, and the posterior chamber could be entered remote from (i.e., peripheral to) the pupil. Not only would a discission *not* be accomplished, but vitreous could present through the peripheral iridectomy. This is the rationale for our choice of the 3 or 9 o'clock incision site for a secondary discission.

Occasionally, there will be a large flap of anterior capsule that adheres to the posterior capsule. This will invariably form an opacity and rarely a fluid-filled cyst. The resultant membrane is tough and difficult to discisse. If an attempt to perform an adequate discission with the hooked needle technique, described previously, is unsuccessful, a two-needle technique may be contemplated. The anterior chamber is entered at the limbus at 3 and 9 o'clock with individual, bent needles, only one of which carries an irrigation line. The other needle is attached to a tuberculin syringe, which acts as a handle. The membrane is perforated in the center with the tip of one needle, and the tip of the second needle is introduced through the perforation site. The needles are simultaneously withdrawn to the pupillary margin, discissing the capsule in two directions simultaneously and avoiding tug by providing countertraction to each other. The needles are turned until the hooks are horizontal and withdrawn from the eye.

Realistically, there are membranes that cannot be perforated and discissed. When these membranes are optically significant, a pars plana membranectomy should be considered. This can be performed without disturbing the IOL. The posterior chamber is entered 3.5 mm posterior to the limbus in the superior temporal quadrant with an automated vitreophage. Infusion can be attained with a cannula placed into the anterior chamber at the limbus in the superior nasal quadrant. With this technique, the vitreophage requires only two functions, cutting and aspiration. Therefore an instrument with a narrower probe may be used, and the sclerotomy will be smaller. The technique is identical to that described for managing pupillary membranes, described next. There are also promising laser techniques being developed for the noninvasive management of posterior capsular opacification.

PUPILLARY MEMBRANE

This is a membrane that bridges the pupillary aperture and may obstruct the visual axis partially or completely (Fig. 9-10). It may occur after an ICCE or an ECCE, but it is classically associated with the former when an interaction occurs between the pupillary margin and the anterior hyaloid face (Fig. 9-11). This results in a membrane that appears and acts like a sec-

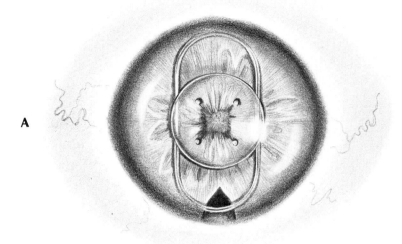

A

Fig. 9-10. A, Pupillary membrane behind a Binkhorst iris clip IOL. **B,** Pupillary membrane behind Copeland IOL, partially occluding the pupil.

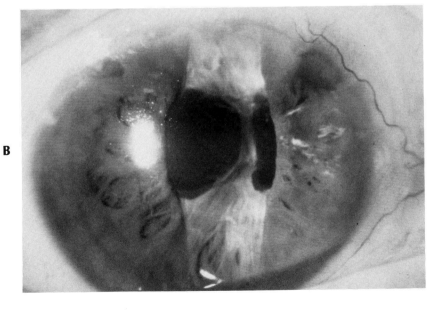

B

ondary cataract and is often amenable to discission as already described (Fig. 9-12). However, these membranes can recur, and when they do, they often contract, pulling the iris centrad and obliterating the pupillary space (Fig. 9-13). A simple discission will not suffice. The recommended treatment is a pars plana vitrectomy approach to remove the anterior vitreous and pupillary membrane (Figs. 9-14 and 9-15). In our experience, these types of membranes are more common with iris-fixated lens implants, especially in those patients maintained with topical miotics.

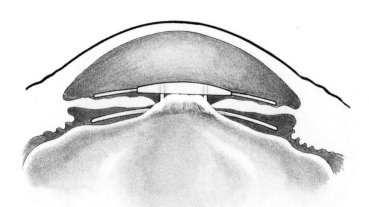

Fig. 9-11. Concept of involvement of anterior hyaloid face in pupillary membrane formation.

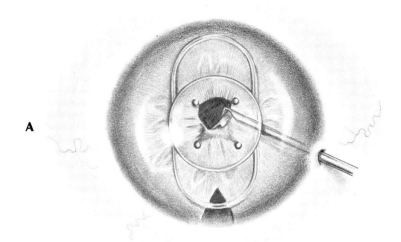

A

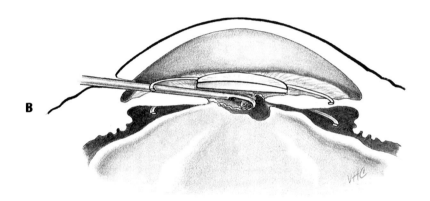

B

Fig. 9-12. A, Discission of a pupillary membrane.
B, Pupillary membrane discission (sagittal view).

Fig. 9-13. Dense retrolental membrane following
an ICCE and Binkhorst iris clip IOL in a patient
who sustained a hypopyon uveitis. (From Jaffe, N.S.,
and others: Pseudophakos, St. Louis, 1978, The
C.V. Mosby Co.)

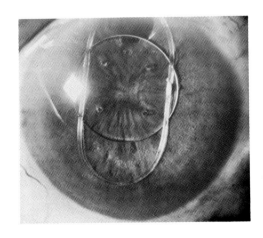

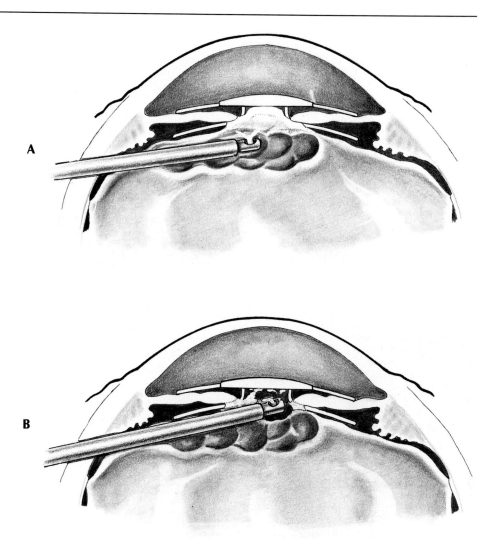

Fig. 9-14. A, Sagittal view of vitreophage removing anterior vitreous as a prelude to a pupillary membranectomy. **B,** Pupillary membrane is engaged and removed by vitreophage. **C,** Appearance of vitreophage tip in pupil resuming its normal form.

C

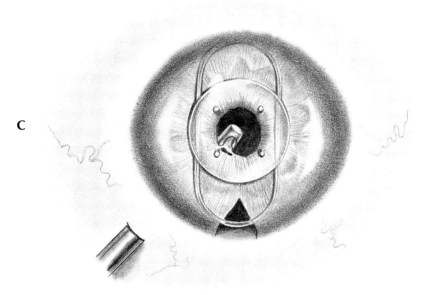

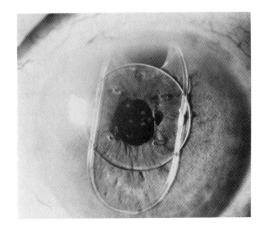

Fig. 9-15. Postoperative appearance of eye shown in Fig. 9-13, following pars plana removal of pupillary membrane. (From Jaffe, N.S., and others: Pseudophakos, St. Louis, 1978, The C.V. Mosby Co.)

RESIDUAL CORTEX

Residual cortex can occlude the visual axis following an ECCE or KPE (Fig. 9-16). As noted previously, the superior capsular cul-de-sac is the area least accessible for cortex removal. Pieces of cortex drop by gravity from this part of the capsular bag and fluff up in the pupil. Other areas of residual cortex also may be culpable. If the patient's vision is unimpaired by this media opacity, we give no treatment except pupillary dilatation, IOL type permitting. For cases in which the visual axis is obstructed, a decision must be made whether to intervene surgically. With observation the cortex may be seen to reabsorb, and for this reason we arbitrarily wait for 6 weeks. Beyond this point, if the cortex persists with no observable improvement, we reoperate. A 3.0-mm incision is made either at the original operative site or in an area of the surgical limbus convenient for the surgeon. The I/A Cooper-Vision Systems/Cavitron handpiece or a vitreophage is inserted into the pupillary aperture (Fig. 9-17), and the residual cortex is aspirated. After having been exposed to the aqueous for several weeks, the cortex is invariably soft and aspirates easily. The handpiece is removed and the incision sutured as required.

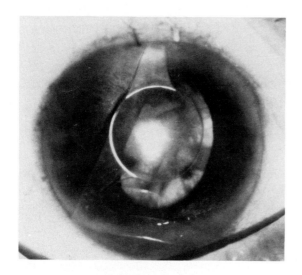

Fig. 9-16. Residual cortex in pupil, following KPE. (Courtesy Dr. Lyle Moses.)

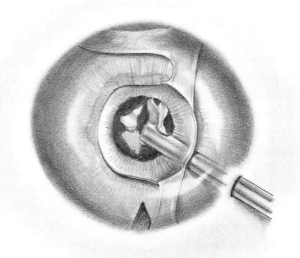

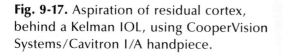

Fig. 9-17. Aspiration of residual cortex, behind a Kelman IOL, using CooperVision Systems/Cavitron I/A handpiece.

VITREOUS HEMORRHAGE

The management of vitreous hemorrhage after IOL surgery is similar to that following routine cataract extraction. The first consideration is the degree of hemorrhage. A minimal hemorrhage requires no treatment. However, a significant vitreous hemorrhage that is optically disabling and persists beyond several weeks is a worrisome problem (Fig. 9-18). Its causes can range from bleeding from the incision, peripheral iridectomy, or ciliary processes, to rhegmatogenous retinal detachment, acute senile macular choroidal degeneration, posterior vitreous separation, or late expulsive hemorrhage. Management of it obviously depends on the cause, and B scan ultrasonography is invaluable in evaluating the diagnosis.

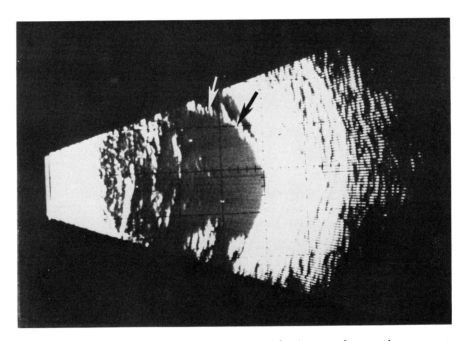

Fig. 9-18. Retinal detachment *(arrows)* in eye with vitreous hemorrhage.

If the only pathologic condition is blood in the posterior chamber, it is reasonable to wait several months before surgical intervention, since many vitreous hemorrhages spontaneously reabsorb. A vitreous hemorrhage clears faster in an aphakic eye than in a phakic eye, and an IOL in situ probably clears it at a rate falling between those two rates. Therefore the next consideration is to determine how long "several months" is; to this, no definitive answer is possible. Certainly we would surgically intervene after 6 months, if the vitreous hemorrhage persists and reduces vision substantially. The surgical procedure would be a pars plana vitrectomy. Retinal detachment is a possible sequela of this operation; therefore the cataract surgeon may prefer to refer these cases to a vitreoretinal specialist. Even though a discussion of vitreous surgery techniques is beyond this book's purposes, we would like to answer the frequently asked question as to which is the best vitreophage. The answer is the one that works with reasonable consistency. When an instrument is used infrequently, operating room personnel are unfamiliar with its maintenance and setup. In contemporary ophthalmology the surgeon is in the hands of high technology, and it is a miserable feeling to be unable to complete a case because of equipment failure.

COMMENTS

In this chapter, we have stressed postoperative media opacities, but the patient's preoperative status impinges on this. Preoperative ocular disorders may confuse the surgeon if it is first diagnosed postoperatively. When the fundus cannot be visualized preoperatively and the patient's history is atypical or unavailable, we advise additional diagnostic tests as appropriate. Fig. 9-19 shows a funnel-shaped retinal detachment on B mode ultrasonography. The patient had a mature cataract in this eye and bilateral posterior synechiae, precluding evaluation of any pupillary afferent defect. It would have been an error to insert an IOL in this case, on the assumption that the cataract was the only cause of vision loss.

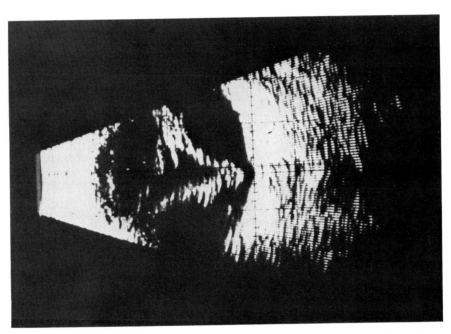

Fig. 9-19. Funnel-shaped retinal detachment in eye with opaque media on B mode ultrasonography.

Ten
Miscellanea

In this chapter we wish to explain points cited in the rest of the text. We wish to discuss further matters either caused by IOL insertion or influencing the decision to implant an IOL.

SODIUM HYALURONATE

In several chapters we have alluded to sodium hyaluronate. Sodium hyaluronate is a transparent viscoelastic substance, which can best be described as vitreous without collagen. It is used in ophthalmology as 1% sodium hyaluronate and 99% water; and although viscous, it adheres neither to glass nor plastic. As a biopolymer, it is found in vitreous and synovial fluid.

The great advantages of sodium hyaluronate can be summed up by stating that its viscosity permits an open chamber to be converted to a closed chamber without the necessity of suturing. For example, consider an ICCE in which positive vitreous pressure obliterates the anterior chamber after cataract extraction. A bolus of sodium hyaluronate reforms the anterior chamber without sutures, and the desired lens implant may be inserted, albeit with the instillation of additional aliquots of sodium hyaluronate as required. In a pseudophakic keratoplasty the iris-pseudophakos diaphragm often bulges forward after the corneal button is removed, and this may place the donor cornea in jeopardy. Sodium hyaluronate, even with an open-sky operative site, will push the iris-pseudophakos diaphragm posteriorly and provide a cushion of viscoelastic fluid between the IOL and donor cornea. In spite of its viscosity, sodium hyaluronate is injectable through a 27-gauge cannula and is completely miscible with all currently available irrigating solutions. Intracameral acetylcholine readily constricts the pupil even though sodium hyaluronate is in the anterior chamber. Sodium hyaluronate can also be used to dilate the pupil by its mechanical bulk. If a pupil is marginal (i.e., a little too large for a miotic pupil technique to be considered [Chapter 7] but too small to hazard an ICCE or impair the anterior capsulectomy with an ECCE or phacoemulsification), then a bolus of sodium hyaluronate, injected intracamerally around the pupillary margin, stretches the pupil. Usually an additional 1 or 2 mm in pupillary dilatation can be obtained.

Sodium hyaluronate has multiple uses in ophthalmology and is especially useful in IOL surgery; yet we do not use it routinely. Idiosyncratic, extremely high intraocular pressures are not infrequent after the use of sodium hyaluronate, and uveitis has been reported following the use of a European brand. Although sodium hyaluronate is completely transparent, it is viscous, and its presence in the anterior chamber can impair the anterior capsulectomy when used in an ECCE or KPE. The reason is that the physical bulk of the substance prevents the anterior capsule from rolling up in a scroll while successive cuts are made in the anterior capsule (pp. 23-24). Notwithstanding these few negative effects, sodium hyaluronate is an extremely important addition to the ophthalmic surgeon's armamentarium.

REMOVAL OF AN IOL

Before we discuss how to remove an IOL, let us consider why an IOL should be removed. An obvious reason is an anterior chamber IOL of incorrect length (p. 228). Not only should this lens be removed, but it also should be replaced with an IOL of correct length. Another reason is an IOL, of whatever type, that dislocates and cannot be securely repositioned. Yet another indication for removal (and replacement if feasible) is an IOL of incorrect power.

A sad era in IOL surgery involved the UGH syndrome (also known as Ellingson's syndrome). This occurred in *injection*-molded anterior chamber IOLs and had two distinct causes. The first involved intracameral warpage of the anterior chamber IOL's feet, so that they assumed a ski-shaped configuration in the angle. The result was intractable uveitis, glaucoma, and hyphema (UGH syndrome), which persisted until the IOL was removed. The second cause of the UGH syndrome was imperfectly finished back surfaces on the IOLs. As these IOLs came out of the mold, small sawlike projections remained on the posterior IOL surface. When the IOL was in situ, physiologic pupillary movements caused the iris to rub against the roughened posterior IOL surface, producing repeated iris excoriations and causing intractable uveitis, glaucoma, and hyphema. The specificity of this syndrome to injection-molded IOLs has been proved by our experience and that of many other surgeons. When the defective IOLs were removed and/or exchanged for equivalent, lathe-cut, *compression*-molded IOLs, the syndrome abruptly abated.

Let us consider how an anterior chamber IOL is removed. This process is the IOL insertion in reverse; every effort should be made to operate on a soft and quiet eye. The pupil should be *constricted* preoperatively and the anterior chamber entered at the initial incision. The incision is opened to a propitious size (7 to 8 mm), and the anterior chamber is formed with either air or sodium hyaluronate. The sclera is retracted over the superior foot or feet; the foot or feet are then grasped by forceps, elevated over the scleral lip of the incision, and externalized. The IOL is withdrawn from the anterior chamber. This method applies to rigid IOLs. The flexible looped IOLs may be enmeshed in the angle, necessitating loop amputation, which has been previously discussed (p. 177).

Analogous to injection-molded IOL problems were problems from the metal-loop era involving iris-fixated IOLs. Facsimiles of the Worst Medallion and Binkhorst iris clip IOLs were manufactured, substituting platinum-iridium or titanium for the plastic loops of the originals. The result was an inordinately heavy IOL with excessive pseudophacodonesis (Fig. 10-1). Many intracapsular cases with these types of metal-looped IOLs exhibited a smoldering uveitis with CME, necessitating IOL removal. It is interesting that the early Binkhorst iridocapsular IOLs (p. 128) had metal loops and gave very acceptable results. We surmise that capsular fixation inhibited pseudophacodonesis.

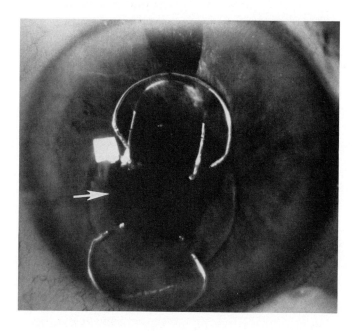

Fig. 10-1. Facsimilie of Binkhorst iris clip IOL, manufactured with metal loops. Lens is excessively heavy and had ruptured pupillary sphincter *(arrow)*. Eye has chronic uveitis.

A two-plane iris-fixated lens is more difficult to remove than a single-plane anterior chamber IOL. As noted with the latter, an iris-fixated IOL is usually removed in a process the reverse of insertion. With an iris-fixated IOL this can involve fixation suture removal (p. 179), dislocation of the loops from behind the iris, and withdrawal of the IOL from the eye. As the lens is removed from the anterior chamber, its two-plane design separates the corneal-scleral incision, enhancing collapse of the anterior chamber. In summary, removal of an iris-fixation IOL offers numerous opportunities for vitreous loss and/or corneal endothelial damage, which could further damage an already compromised eye.

Indications for removal of correctly positioned iridocapsular and posterior chamber IOLs are rare. This is just as well, because capsular fixation of the optic or fibrosis of the capsule to the loops makes removal a technically difficult task. Attempts can be made to lyse the adhesions between the capsule and IOL with a spatula, but this may not be successful, and the IOL may have to be dissected free with microscissors (e.g., Vannas scissors). There is, of course, the risk of capsular rupture and vitreous loss. On the rare occasions on which we have removed lenses of these types, we have found that a sector iridectomy over the superior loop allows visualization and estimation of the amount of capsular-IOL fibrosis present and facilitates IOL removal. Occasionally the lens has to be removed piecemeal, i.e., the loops are amputated from the optic, which is removed, and then all or some of the loops are extracted. Sodium hyaluronate is invaluable in these cases. The reader may ask what the rare indications are for removing well-fixated iridocapsular or posterior chamber IOLs. In our experience, these are, first, the necessity to visualize the posterior segment, second, intractable uveitis, and third, incorrect IOL power.

Another frequently asked question is how to manage the IOL that has completely dislocated into the posterior chamber. These lenses usually come to rest on the peripheral retina at the 6 o'clock position and become adherent to the tissue. To remove such lenses is an invitation for a retinal tear; they are best left alone, and the patient fitted with a contact lens. A lens that is floating in the vitreous can sometimes be prolapsed into the anterior chamber by placing the patient prone and dilating the pupil with a short-acting mydriatic. If the lens floats anteriorly and the pupil then constricts, the IOL will be trapped in the anterior chamber. The surgeon has the option of repositioning the dislocated IOL or removing it. The latter is desirable, if the IOL has a propensity to dislocate and cannot be sutured to the iris.

The cases in which the dislocated IOL is neither adherent to the peripheral retina nor mobile enough to prolapse into the anterior chamber present a vexing problem. If the lens is in the posterior chamber but floating in the anterior vitreous, it is frequently possible to secure one of the haptic loops with a microhook (e.g., Hirschman hook) passed through a limbal incision. The IOL is then drawn into the anterior chamber, where it is repositioned or removed, as already noted. The surgeon may have to perform an anterior vitrectomy, for which an automated vitreophage is preferred. Of course, this technique presupposes the availability of a haptic loop that can be hooked with the instrument. One-piece IOLs, such as the Choyce (p. 56), Kelman (p. 68), Copeland (p. 114), and others, are not amenable to this technique. For these lenses, and for cases in which the dislocated IOL is in the middle or posterior vitreous, the surgeon must decide whether to observe the IOL in the hope that it will settle and adhere to ocular tissue or intervene surgically.

The latter will necessitate a pars plana incision with a two- or three-portal approach. The lens is secured with an instrument such as Neubauer vitreous forceps and brought anteriorly, as the adherent or impeding vitreous is removed with a vitreophage. To remove the IOL through the pars plana is probably unwise, because the sclerotomy might have to be enlarged to 8 mm or more, depending on the IOL type, with the attendant risk of retinal dialysis and detachment as the IOL is manipulated through the sclerotomy. We feel it is preferable to pass the IOL anteriorly through the pupil and remove it through a limbal section (or reposition it). These cases can be formidable, and operative or postoperative retinal holes or detachment is always a possibility. For this reason, a referral to a vitreoretinal surgeon may be desirable. This type of dislocation was seen most frequently in unsutured iris-fixated IOLs. With declining usage of these lenses, it is hoped that this type of complication will become rare.

SHEETS GLIDE

This is a 3- to 4-mm wide strip of thin plastic, which has multiple uses in anterior segment surgery, a few of which have now been made obsolete by the availability of sodium hyaluronate. The glide is particularly useful in IOLs designed to be placed in the capsular bag, specifically during the placement of the inferior IOL loop (Fig. 10-2). The glide is passed into the anterior chamber so that its advancing edge passes through the pupillary aperture, under the inferior capsular flap, and into the inferior capsular cul-de-sac. The IOL is then introduced into the anterior chamber and slid down the glide, which directs the inferior loop into the inferior cul-de-sac. (We liken this to one's heel being guided into a shoe by a shoehorn.) The IOL is steadied as the glide is withdrawn from the anterior chamber, and the superior loop is positioned. Sometimes the superior iris is retracted peripherally as the glide is being withdrawn, and the superior loop merely drops into position fortuitously; but the surgeon should not count on this.

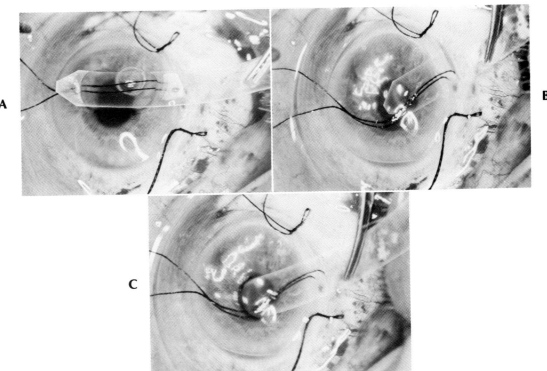

Fig. 10-2. A, Sheets glide prior to insertion. **B,** Glide advancing into anterior chamber. **C,** Glide in situ with tip under inferior iris. (From Jaffe, N.S., and others: Pseudophakos, St. Louis, 1978, The C.V. Mosby Co.)

The Sheets glide is useful in KPE and ECCE. For example in a KPE, positive vitreous pressure and anterior chamber collapse may inhibit the insertion of the ultrasonic probe into the anterior chamber (p. 42). The iris rises to block the incision, and the probe plows into the iris as attempts are made to advance it across the superior iris. The surgeon's persistence will be met with an iridodialysis and possible hemorrhage. A Sheets glide will bridge the iris and provide a smooth surface, along which the probe can be safely inserted. Another use is during the I/A phase (p. 31) of either an ECCE or KPE, when the capsule is inadvertently ruptured. In these cases the CooperVision Systems/Cavitron unit should be placed in I/A minimum and the irrigating bottle lowered. The capsular rupture can be bridged with the glide while additional cortex is aspirated. In an ICCE in which there is positive vitreous pressure after cataract extraction, a Sheets glide may be used to facilitate IOL insertion. The corneal-scleral section should be closed to leave an 8-mm unsutured area of incision superiorly. The pupil is constricted with acetylcholine, and air is instilled into the anterior chamber. The Sheets glide is slid into the anterior chamber under the air bubble and *over* the inferior iris, if an anterior chamber IOL is to be inserted. The IOL is then introduced into the anterior chamber and slid along the glide, which bridges the pupil and the anterior hyaloid face. The Sheets glide guides the inferior feet of the IOL into the inferior angle. The IOL is steadied as the glide is slowly withdrawn, and the body of the IOL bridges the pupil and anterior hyaloid face. Additional aliquots of air are added as required, and the superior feet are positioned (p. 60).

For an iris-fixated IOL such as the Binkhorst iris clip, the Sheets glide is slid *under* the inferior iris. The cornea is retracted slightly, and the IOL is slid into the anterior chamber and along the glide, with a slight posterior pressure against it. This will push the anterior hyaloid face posteriorly and create a negative pressure within the anterior chamber, which preserves the air bubble and may encourage the passage of more air into the anterior chamber. The glide guides the posterior inferior loop behind the inferior iris, at which point the glide is withdrawn. As noted before, the withdrawal of the glide may retract the superior iris, permitting the superior posterior loop to drop behind the superior iris. If this does not occur, the superior loops are positioned after the glide is withdrawn from the eye. Sodium hyaluronate has largely obviated the need for a Sheets glide as an adjunct to intracapsular surgery.

IOLS AND GLAUCOMA

In Chapter 7 we discussed the surgical techniques required for managing the miotic pupil in conjunction with IOL surgery. The most common reason for miosis in a clinical surgical practice is chronic miotic therapy in glaucoma patients who subsequently require cataract surgery. The point we wish to ponder here is whether glaucoma patients should have IOLs. There is no agreement on this in the ophthalmologic profession, but we shall state our opinion: it depends on the control of the intraocular pressure. For example, a patient who has glaucoma without progression of field loss or disc/cup ratio and who is well controlled with topical medication is a candidate for IOL surgery. On the other hand, the patient with unsatisfactory intraocular pressure, field loss, and progressive disc changes requires laser and/or glaucoma surgery as an initial procedure because the glaucoma takes precedence over the cataract.

If the result of laser or glaucoma surgery is satisfactory, can the patient have an IOL? We would say yes, but many surgeons would not. Our preference is to wait several months and then perform cataract surgery with IOL insertion from an incision remote from the bleb, if a filtering procedure was used as the initial operation. Specifically, we would perform a superior trabeculectomy as the first operation, followed by a temporal section for the cataract/IOL surgery. Actually, the trabeculectomy is best performed in the superior nasal quadrant, which permits a true temporal section for the cataract extraction. When a trabeculectomy is performed at the 12 o'clock position, and filtration occurs, the resultant bleb usually spreads laterally. The temporal cataract section then becomes an inferior temporal section in an effort to avoid the bleb at the superior aspect of the incision (Fig. 10-3). The surgeon should remember that anterior chamber IOLs (Chapter 2) require access to an angle free from peripheral anterior synechiae, which may appear after a filtering procedure if the anterior chamber shallowed for several days.

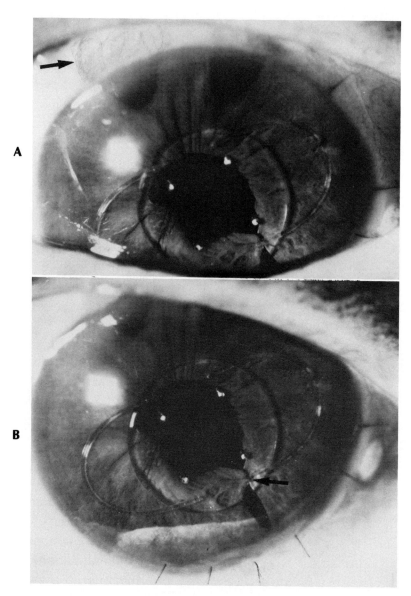

Fig. 10-3. A, Binkhorst iris clip IOL inserted into eye with previous filtering surgery. Note superior bleb *(arrow)*. **B,** Same eye; note inferior iridoplasty *(arrow)* and inferior temporal section.

IOLS AND VITREOUS LOSS

Should an IOL be inserted after vitreous loss? This is also extremely controversial. We generally would insert an IOL, but this view is vigorously opposed by many experienced IOL surgeons. Our opinion is based on our contention that the subsequent fate of the eye is independent of the IOL's presence. When we perform intracapsular surgery and lose vitreous while delivering the cataract or inserting the IOL, we perform an anterior vitrectomy and proceed thereafter with the IOL insertion. Our initial maneuver is an attempt to aspirate liquid vitreous, which if successful often suffices (Fig. 10-4). If liquid vitreous cannot be aspirated, the anterior vitrectomy is performed with an automated vitreophage, until the iris is concave, and an air bubble is pulled into the anterior chamber by the negative pressure created by the vitreous removal; then the IOL is inserted.

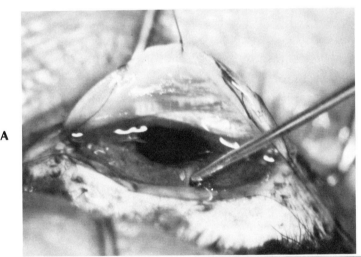

A

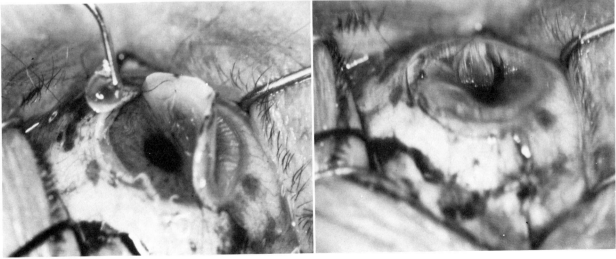

B   C

Fig. 10-4. A, Needle inserted into posterior chamber through peripheral iridectomy. **B,** Aspiration of liquid vitreous. **C,** Collapsed globe after vitreous aspiration. (From Jaffe, N.S.: Cataract surgery and its complications, ed. 3, St. Louis, 1981, The C.V. Mosby Co.)

In the Binkhorst iris clip IOL technique, vitreous is sometimes lost at the peripheral iridectomy during passage of the transiridectomy suture (p. 96). We find this to be of no clinical significance, and merely remove the presenting vitreous with cellulose sponges and a scissor excision, taking care that no vitreous wick remains in the wound. Sometimes, after no vitreous loss has been noticed at surgery, vitreous is seen postoperatively in the anterior chamber, prolapsing through the pupil or peripheral iridectomy. This, too, is clinically insignificant.

Vitreous loss in conjunction with extracapsular cataract surgery presents some additional problems. First, a J-loop posterior chamber IOL cannot safely be left in situ if there has been a large rupture of the posterior capsule; thus its insertion should not be attempted. Another type of IOL should be selected. Our preference is an anterior chamber IOL, although an iris clip model also suffices. Then there is the management of the vitreous itself, which ranges from no management at all to an automated vitrectomy with aspiration of residual cortex. For example, if there is capsular rupture at the conclusion of the irrigation/aspiration phase of the operation, with aspiration of minimal vitreous that quickly falls back into the posterior chamber, then no further vitrectomy is required. However, if a capsule ruptures before the bulk of the cortex has been removed, and there is significant vitreous loss with unformed vitreous mixing with cortex, an automated anterior vitrectomy should be performed to remove both vitreous and cortex as well as any capsule that may obscure the pupillary aperture.

A calamitous occurrence is capsular rupture with vitreous loss and posterior dislocation of the nucleus into the vitreous cavity. An anterior automated vitrectomy should be performed to remove the vitreous from the anterior chamber and any residual cortex. If balanced saline is instilled to reform the chamber, the surgeon may be lucky enough to have the nucleus float anteriorly, where it can be removed with either a cryoprobe or a loop. Most dislocated nuclei do not oblige in this fashion, and we advise closing the eye and observing the case, albeit with topical and systemic corticosteroid therapy. A *minority* of eyes will recuperate without any further intervention, but most will require a pars plana approach either to manipulate the nucleus into the anterior chamber from which it is removed or, in the case of a soft nucleus, to remove it completely. For the anterior segment surgeon unfamiliar with these techniques, we recommend referral of the patient to a vitreoretinal surgeon.

SECONDARY IOL IMPLANTATION

A secondary IOL refers to an implantation remote from the original cataract surgery, i.e., the insertion of an IOL into an eye rendered aphakic by prior cataract extraction. In this state, if the eye previously had a KPE or ECCE with an intact posterior capsule, then any type of IOL may be secondarily inserted. If in the previous cataract extraction a discission was performed, then posterior chamber IOL implantation would probably be technically difficult, and we would select another type of IOL.

In eyes where an ICCE was the initial procedure, only an iris-fixated or anterior chamber IOL can be inserted. The problem with ICCE cases is how to manage vitreous in the anterior chamber, and there is no consensus on this. Opinions range from believing that any vitreous in the anterior chamber contraindicates secondary IOL implantation to ignoring the vitreous completely. We think that the truth is in between. If the anterior chamber is full of vitreous, we think it is poor judgment to ignore it and/or perform a vitrectomy to insert an IOL secondarily, except in unusual circumstances. However, a small amount of vitreous in the anterior chamber does not contraindicate secondary IOL insertion.

Irrespective of the type of cataract extraction, we unreservedly state that secondary IOL implantation is easier with a single-plane IOL. If the posterior capsule is intact, we insert a J-loop posterior chamber IOL (Chapter 5). If the capsule has been discissed or in ICCE cases, we insert an anterior chamber IOL.

When a posterior chamber IOL is to be inserted as a secondary IOL implantation, the pupil should be moderately dilated. The lens may be inserted by reopening the original incision or by means of a temporal section, which is our preference because it avoids snagging the peripheral iridectomies from the initial surgery. For the same reason, if an anterior chamber IOL is secondarily inserted, we also advocate a temporal incision (Fig. 10-5).

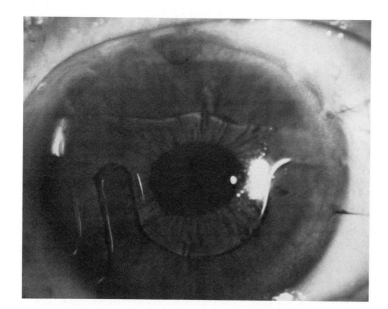

Fig. 10-5. Kelman anterior chamber IOL horizontally in situ following a secondary implantation through a temporal incision.

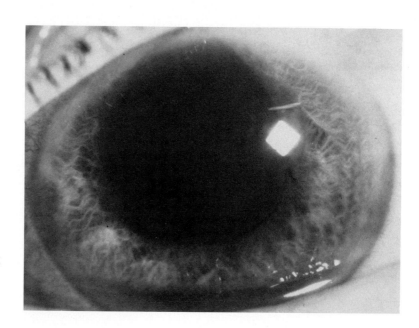

Fig. 10-6. Peaked pupil following posterior chamber KPE and insertion of posterior chamber IOL.

CONCLUSION

In this book, we have not discussed all IOLs nor all conceivable techniques. We have tried to provide guidance to methods adaptable by most surgeons, always aware that cataract surgery and intraocular lens implantation will continue to evolve.

We would remind the reader that the complications of IOL surgery are all the complications of cataract surgery plus the complications caused by insertion and intraocular presence of the IOL. Fig. 10-6 shows a patient who had a posterior chamber phacoemulsification with the insertion of a posterior chamber IOL. The pupil is peaked superiorly. Inspection of the wound showed a knuckle of prolapsed iris between two sutures (Fig. 10-7). Thus, in spite of a modern and sophisticated technique, a classic complication of cataract surgery occurred. Notwithstanding the best of intentions and abilities, some complications are inevitable. The surgeon can keep them to a minimum by meticulously attending to technique and using IOLs of impeccable quality.

In the future, we predict that IOL implantation will be prescribed for the majority of adult patients for whom cataract surgery is contemplated.

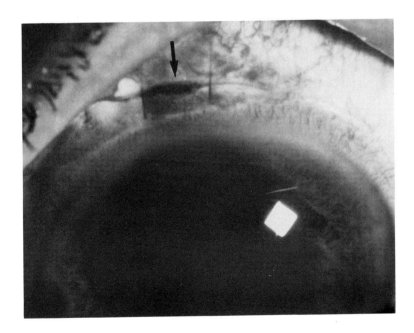

Fig. 10-7. Same case as shown in Fig. 10-6. Note iris prolapse *(arrow)*.

Bibliography

Alpar, J.J.: Cataract extraction and lens implantation in eyes with preexisting filtering blebs, J. Am. Intraocul. Implant Soc. **5**:33, 1979.

Beckman, H.: Bending of excessively long intraocular suture material by argon laser, Am. J. Ophthalmol. **91**:401, 1981.

Binkhorst, C.D.: The iridocapsular (two-loop) lens and the iris-clip (four-loop) lens in pseudophakia, Trans. Am. Acad. Ophthalmol. Otolaryngol. **77**:589, 1973.

Binkhorst, C.D.: Evaluation of intraocular lens fixation in pseudophakia. Am. J. Ophthalmol. **80**:184, 1975.

Binkhorst, C.D.: Five hundred planned extracapsular extractions with iridocapsular and iris clip lens implantation in senile cataract, Ophthalmic Surg. **8**:37, 1977.

Binkhorst, C.D.: Advantages and disadvantages of intracameral Na-hyaluronate in intraocular lens surgery, Doc. Ophthalmol. **50**:233, 1981.

Binkhorst, C.D.: Cataract extraction and intraocular lens implantation after fistulizing glaucoma surgery, J. Am. Intraocul. Implant Soc. **7**:133, 1981.

Bourne, W.M., Brubaker, R.F., and O'Fallon, W.M.: Use of air to decrease endothelial cell loss during intraocular lens implantation, Arch. Ophthalmol. **97**:1473, 1979.

Bourne, W.M., and others: Corneal trauma in intracapsular and extracapsular cataract extraction with lens implantation, Arch. Ophthalmol. **99**:1375, 1981.

Choyce, D.P.: Intraocular lenses and implants, London, 1964, H.K. Lewis & Co. Ltd.

Choyce, D.P.: The Choyce Mark VIII anterior chamber implant: primary and secondary implantation compared, Ophthalmic Surg. **8**:49, 1977.

Choyce, D.P.: The Choyce Mark VIII and Mark IX anterior chamber implants, J. Am. Intraocul. Implant Soc. **5**:217, 1979.

Choyce, D.P.: The evolution of the anterior chamber implant up to, and including, the Choyce Mark IX, Ophthalmology **86**:197, 1979.

Clayman, H.M.: Lens implant forceps, Trans. Am. Acad. Ophthalmol. Otolaryngol. **83**:853, 1977.

Clayman, H.M.: Technique for insertion of the superior loop of the Shearing-style posterior chamber lens, J. Am. Intraocul. Implant Soc. **4**:383, 1980.

Clayman, H.M.: The trend in intraocular lens implantation (editorial), J. Am. Intraocul. Implant Soc. **6**:15, 1980.

Clayman, H.M., Jaffe, N.S., and Light, D.S.: Lens implantation and diabetes mellitus, Am. J. Ophthalmol. **88**:990, 1979.

Clayman, H.M., and others: Lens implantation, miosis, and glaucoma, Am. J. Ophthalmol. **87**:121, 1979.

Clayman, H.M., and others: Intraocular lenses, axial length, and retinal detachment, Am. J. Ophthalmol. **92**:778, 1981.

Cohan, B.E.: Broken nylon iris-fixation suture, Am. J. Ophthalmol. **93**:507, 1982.

Cohan, B.E., Pearch, A.C., and Schwartz, S.: Broken nylon iris-fixation sutures, Am. J. Ophthalmol. **88**:982, 1979.

Drews, R.C.: Lens implantation in patients with glaucoma, Ophthalmology **87**:665, 1980.

Drews, R.C.: The Pearce tripod posterior chamber intraocular lens: an independent analysis of Pearce's results, J. Am. Intraocul. Implant Soc. **6**:259, 1980.

Drews, R.C.: The medallion lens five years later, J. Am. Intraocul. Implant Soc. **7**:49, 1981.

Dulaney, D.D., and Maloney, W.F.: Technique for closed-chamber insertion of transiridectomy prolene clip lens, J. Am. Intraocul. Implant Soc. **4**:8, 1978.

Ellingson, F.T.: The uveitis-glaucoma-hyphema syndrome associated with the Mark VIII anterior chamber lens implant, J. Am. Intraocul. Implant Soc. **4**:50, 1978.

Emery, J.E., and Little, J.H.: Phacoemulsification and aspiration of cataracts: surgical techniques, complications, and results, St. Louis, 1979, The C.V. Mosby Co.

Fechner, P.U.: Laser-coagulation of ruptured fixation suture after lens implantation, J. Am. Intraocul. Implant Soc. **4**:54, 1978.

Fine, M.: Keratoplasty for bullous keratoplasty with intraocular lens, J. Am. Intraocul. Implant Soc. **4**:12, 1978.

Forstot, S.L., and others: The effect of intraocular lens implantation on the corneal endothelium, Trans. Am. Acad. Ophthalmol. Otolaryngol. **83**:195, 1977.

Galin, M.A., Poole, T.A., and Obstbaum, S.A.: Retinal detachment in pseudophakia, Am. J. Ophthalmol. **88**:49, 1979.

Galin, M.A., and others: Time analysis of corneal endothelial cell density after cataract extraction, Am. J. Ophthalmol. **88**:93, 1979.

Graether, J.M.: A new method of inserting the J-loop posterior chamber lens to achieve capsular fixation and consistent centering, J. Am. Intraocul. Implant Soc. **7**:70, 1981.

Hamdi, T.N.: The Copeland intraocular lens: five to ten years later, Ophthalmology **86**:984, 1979.

Heslin, K.B.: Is "white-to-white" right? J. Am. Intraocul. Implant Soc. **5**:50, 1979.

Jaffe, N.S.: Cataract surgery: a modern attitude toward a technological explosion, N. Engl. J. Med. **299**:235, 1978.

Jaffe, N.S.: Results of intraocular lens implant surgery: the third Binkhorst medal lecture, Am. J. Ophthalmol. **85**:13, 1978.

Jaffe, N.S.: Cataract surgery and its complications, ed. 3, St. Louis, 1981, The C.V. Mosby Co.

Jaffe, N.S., and others: A comparison of 500 Binkhorst implants with 500 routine intracapsular cataract extractions, Am. J. Ophthalmol. **85**:24, 1978.

Jaffe, N.S., and others: Pseudophakos, St. Louis, 1978, The C.V. Mosby Co.

Jaffe, N.S., and others: Dislocation of Binkhorst four-loop lens implant, Ophthalmology **86**:207, 1979.

Jaffe, N.S., and others: The results of intracapsular cataract extraction with a Binkhorst iris clip lens implant 34 to 40 months after surgery, Ophthalmic Surg. **11**:489, 1980.

Jaffe, N.S., and others: The results of lens implantation in eyes with operative loss of vitreous, J. Am. Intraocul. Implant Soc. **6**:243, 1980.

Jungschaffer, O.H.: Retinal detachment after intraocular lens implants, Arch. Ophthalmol. **95**:1203, 1977.

Keates, R.H., and Lichtenstein, S.B.: Surgical complications of Choyce-type implants, Ophthalmology **86**:625, 1979.

Keates, R.H., and Lichtenstein, S.B.: The Kelman and other anterior chamber lenses, Ophthalmic Surg. **11**:708, 1980.

Kelman, C.D.: Phacoemulsification and aspiration: the Kelman technique of cataract removal, New York, 1975, Aesculapius Publishing, Inc.

Knolle, G.E., Jr.: Bending the platinum clip, J. Am. Intraocul. Implant Soc. **5**:61, 1979.

Kokoris, N., and Macy, J.I.: Laser iridectomy of acute pseudophakic pupillary block glaucoma, J. Am. Intraocul. Implant Soc. **8**:33, 1982.

Kraff, M.C., Sanders, D.R., and Lieberman, H.L.: The medallion suture lens: management of complications, Ophthalmology **86**:643, 1979.

Kraff, M.C., Sanders, D.R., and Lieberman, N.L.: 300 primary anterior chamber lens implantations: gonioscopic findings and specular microscopy, J. Am. Intraocul. Implant Soc. **5**:207, 1979.

Kraff, M.C., Sanders, D.R., and Lieberman, H.L.: Specular microscopy in cataract and intraocular lens patients: a report of 564 cases, Arch. Ophthalmol. **98**:1782, 1980.

Kratz, R.P., and others: A comparative analysis of anterior chamber, iris-supported, capsule-fixated, and posterior chamber intraocular lenses following cataract extraction by phacoemulsification, Ophthalmology **88**:56, 1981.

Kratz, R.P., and others: The Shearing intraocular lens: a report of 1,000 cases, J. Am. Intraocul. Implant Soc. **7**:55, 1981.

Kronenthal, R.L.: Nylon in the anterior chamber, Ophthalmology **88**:965, 1981.

Kwitko, M.L.: The Fyodorov Sputnik intraocular lens, Ophthalmology **86**:638, 1979.

Kwitko, M.L.: The platinum clip (Platina) intraocular lens, Ophthalmology **86**:632, 1979.

Little, J.: Outline of phacoemulsification for the ophthalmic surgeon, ed. 2, Oklahoma City, 1975, Semco Color Press.

Makley, T.R., and Keates, R.H.: Detachment of Descemet's membrane with insertion of an intraocular lens, Ophthalmic Surg. **11**:492, 1980.

McCannel, M.A.: A retrievable suture idea for anterior uveal problems, Ophthalmic Surg. **7**:98, 1976.

McIntyre, D.J.: The McCannel suture: a bimanual technique, J. Am. Intraocul. Implant Soc. **5**:151, 1979.

Meyer, R.F., and Sugar, A.: Penetrating keratoplasty in pseudophakic bullous keratopathy, Am. J. Ophthalmol. **90**: 677, 1980.

Miami Study Group: Cystoid macular edema in aphakic and pseudophakic eyes, Am. J. Ophthalmol. **88**:45, 1979.

Miller, D., and Stegmann, R.: Use of Na-hyaluronate in anterior segment eye surgery, J. Am. Intraocul. Implant Soc. **6**:13, 1980.

Miller, D., and Stegmann, R.: Use of sodium hyaluronate in human IOL implantation, Ann. Ophthalmol. **13**:811, 1981.

Moses, L.: Pupillary-block glaucoma after Choyce lens implantation, J. Am. Intraocul. Implant Soc. **4**:50, 1978.

Murphy, G.E.: A technique for suturing the Shearing posterior chamber implant to the iris, J. Am. Intraocul. Implant Soc. **7**:167, 1981.

Nordlohne, M.E.: The intraocular implant lens: development and results with special reference to the Binkhorst lens, The Hague, 1975, Dr. W. Junk BV, Publishers,

Obstbaum, S.A.: Management of glaucoma in the implanted patient, J. Am. Intraocul. Implant Soc. **7**:252, 1981.

Obstbaum, S.A., and others: Laser photomydriasis in pseudophakic pupillary block, J. Am. Intraocul. Implant Soc. **7**: 28, 1981.

Oglesby, R.B.: Complications of the Copeland implant, Ophthalmology **86**:667, 1979.

Olson, R.J., Morgan, K.S., and Kolodner, H.: The Shearing-style intraocular lens and the posterior chamber, J. Am. Intraocul. Implant Soc. **5**:338, 1979.

Olson, R.J., and others: Refractive variation and donor tissue size in aphakic keratoplasty, Arch. Ophthalmol. **97**:1480, 1979.

Pape, L.G.: Intracapsular and extracapsular techniques of lens implantation with Healon, J. Am. Intraocul. Implant Soc. **6**:342, 1980.

Pearce, J.L.: Pearce-style posterior chamber lenses, J. Am. Intraocul. Implant Soc. **6**:33, 1980.

Polack, F.M., Demong, T., and Santaella, H.: Sodium hyaluronate (Healon) in keratoplasty and IOL implantation, Ophthalmology **88**:425, 1981.

Ruiz, R.S., and Teeters, V.W.: The vitreous wick syndrome: a late complication following cataract surgery, Am. J. Ophthalmol. **70**:483, 1970.

Sheets, J.H., and Maida, J.W.: Lens glide in implant surgery, Arch. Ophthalmol. **96**:145, 1978.

Shepard, D.D.: The fate of eyes from which intraocular lenses have been removed, Ophthalmic Surg. **10**:58, 1979.

Simcoe, C.W.: Simcoe posterior chamber lens: theory, technique and results, J. Am. Intraocul. Implant Soc. **7**:154, 1981.

Sinskey, R.M., and Cain, W., Jr.: The posterior capsule and phacoemulsification, J. Am. Intraocul. Implant Soc. **4**: 206, 1978.

Stark, W.J., Bruner, W.E., and Michels, R.G.: Management of retropseudophakos membranes, J. Am. Intraocul. Implant Soc. **6**:137, 1980.

Taylor, D.M., Khaliq, A., and Maxwell, R.: Keratoplasty and intraocular lenses: current status, Ophthalmology **86**:242, 1979.

Thorburn, D.E., and Levenson, J.E.: Corneal endothelial damage from previously implanted intraocular lenses, J. Am. Intraocul. Implant Soc. **6**:236, 1980.

Wilkinson, C.P.: Retinal detachments following intraocular lens implantation, Ophthalmology **88**:410, 1981.

Index